Manual of Nephrology

Drug Therapy and Therapeutic Protocols in Renal Diseases

Momir Macanovic and Peter Mathieson

Universal Publishers
Boca Raton, Florida
USA • 2005

Manual of Nephrology:
Drug Therapy and Therapeutic Protocols in Renal Diseases

Copyright © 2004 Momir Macanovic and Peter Mathieson
All rights reserved.

Universal Publishers
Boca Raton, Florida
USA • 2005

ISBN: 1-58112-516-X

www.universal-publishers.com

DISCLAIMER

This manual contains protocols and guidance documents assembled by the authors during many years of clinical experience in nephrology. Many are not evidence-based but we have found them useful and hope that others will do likewise. All treatments must remain at the discretion of the physician responsible for the patient's care and we can accept no responsibility for the outcomes.

The recommendations were made on the basis of clinical trials wherever possible. In the absence of relevant clinical trials, we used evidence available or our personal experience.

Our aim was to provide a manual for the treatment of the most frequent kidney diseases or disorders related to the practice of Nephrology. The information may be of use to nephrologists, general internists, general practitioners or medical students.

For more comprehensive discussions readers are referred to the more extensive textbooks, some of them were cited in the references.

GLOSSARY, ABBREVIATIONS

ACEI: angiotensin converting enzyme inhibitor
AF: atrial fibrillation
APD: automated peritoneal dialysis
APTT: activated partial thromboplastin time
AIIRA: angiotensin II receptor antagonist
ARF: acute renal failure
BD: twice daily
BSA: body surface area
CAPD: continuous ambulatory peritoneal dialysis
COPD: chronic obstructive pulmonary disease
COX: cyclo-oxygenase
CRF: chronic renal failure
CVP: central venous pressure
D: day
DNA: deoxyribonucleic acid
DVT: deep vein thrombosis
FBC: full blood count
FFP: fresh frozen plasma
HD: haemodialysis
IM: intramuscular
INR: international normalised ratio
IP: intra-peritoneal
IV: intravenous
LFTs: liver function tests
MI: myocardial infarction
MRSA: methicillin resistant staphylococcus aureus
NSAID: non-steroidal anti-inflammatory drug
OD: once daily
PCWP: pulmonary capillary wedge pressure
PD: peritoneal dialysis

PE: pulmonary embolism
PO: per os (oral administration)
PR: per rectum
PT: prothrombin time
QDS: four times per day
RF: renal failure
RI: renal insufficiency
rHuEpo: recombinant human erythropoietin
SC: subcutaneous
TPN: total parenteral nutrition
TDS: three times per day
U: unit(s)

ACIDOSIS (METABOLIC ACIDOSIS IN CHRONIC RENAL FAILURE, CRF)

Treatment of metabolic acidosis in CRF with sodium bicarbonate is usually well tolerated, i.e. no increase in sodium retention, no oedema and no hypertension. The aim of the treatment is to maintain plasma bicarbonate > 22 mmol/l. The amount of administered sodium bicarbonate should be appropriate to the bicarbonate deficit and it can be administered as:

- Intravenously (unless fluid overload is also present), 1.26% isotonic sodium bicarbonate 500 ml or 1000 ml IV infusion (give an amount appropriate to the bicarbonate deficit).
- Orally, in chronic metabolic acidosis sodium bicarbonate can be given as 600 mg capsules or 500 mg tablets up to 3 g/d PO
- The best method to correct metabolic acidosis in patients on dialysis is to increase dialysate bicarbonate concentration up to 40 mmol/l
- In an emergency, 8.4% sodium bicarbonate solution (50 mmol) 50 ml IV over 30 min or 1 ml/kg body weight can be used, but 1.26% sodium bicarbonate is preferable because of the danger of overdosing.

ACUTELY DISTURBED PATIENT

- Haloperidol may be given orally in a range of 1.5 to 3 mg bd to tds. The IM or IV dose is 2 to 10 mg depending on the clinical manifestations and should be adjusted according to response.
- Diazepam 2 to 5 mg orally (preferably) is the alternative; it can be given parenterally up to 10 mg IM or as slow IV infusion. Parenteral use must be with caution as respiratory depression can occur. The reversal agent Flumazenil should be available.

ACUTE RENAL FAILURE (ARF)

The aetiology should be sought and if possible identified in order to apply specific treatment for prerenal hypovolemia, specific parenchymal renal disease or post renal obstruction. Ultrasound scan of kidneys and bladder may exclude acute on chronic renal failure or post renal obstruction. If intrinsic renal parenchymal disease is suspected as a cause of ARF and if the diagnosis of acute tubular necrosis is not clear from clinical presentation, renal biopsy should be done (may be urgent, and urgent transfer to a specialist renal unit should be considered). Heavy proteinuria and/or haematuria on dipstick testing of the urine suggest glomerular disease. Urgent serological tests for systemic diseases that can present with ARF should be undertaken (eg anti-neutrophil cytoplasm autoantibody, ANCA, for small vessel vasculitis; anti-glomerular basement membrane antibodies for Goodpasture's disease; anti-double stranded DNA antibodies for systemic lupus erythematosus; serum complement C3 and C4 for immune complex disease or complement deficiency). However, if clinical features are suggestive, specialist renal advice should be sought without waiting for results of these laboratory investigations.

Pre-renal ARF requires aggressive correction of hypovolaemia with fluid replacement. The volume of replacement fluid = previous 24 h urine output + estimated loss of fluid by diarrhoea, vomiting etc. + insensible loss (500 ml, more if febrile or in hot climate). Colloid or crystalloid solutions may be used to achieve normovolaemia confirmed by clinical signs and central venous pressure (CVP). The choice of replacement fluid should ideally be guided by information about the type(s) of fluid lost. Remember that loss of water alone is uncommon so that dextrose solutions alone are rarely adequate for replacement: some additional salt is usually required.

In patients with volume depletion begin with 500 mL of isotonic saline IV within 30 – 60 minutes. Repeat infusion of the same volume once or twice until urine output of 1 – 2 mL/min is achieved and then give IV fluid on basis of urine output. Measure central venous pressure CVP (if possible).

Diuretics do not prevent acute renal failure and the role of dopamine is very controversial. In the early phase of ARF, assuming

hypovolemia has been corrected; an oliguric patient may be given one of the diuretics:
- Frusemide bolus 40–250 mg slowly IV or 10-40 mg/hour IV infusion. This may increase urine volume to a useful extent but should not be repeated if it fails to do so.
- Bumetanide 1 mg PO/IV or
- Torasemide 5-40 mg PO.

Catheterization for assessment of hourly urine output is necessary. Take out catheter as soon as oliguria confirmed. The catheter is a source of infection.

Renal dose of dopamine 2–5 µg/kg/min IV is still controversial.

Pulmonary oedema, acidosis and/or hyperkalaemia not responsive to conservative treatment may require dialysis (see also "Hyperkalaemia"). Dialysis options are:
- One of many varieties of continuous renal replacement therapies
- Haemodialysis (daily or alternate day)
- Peritoneal dialysis

Choice of treatment is dependent upon various factors including availability, expertise of staff, haemodynamic stability of the patient, vascular access; whether the primary need is fluid removal or solute removal or both, etc.

Treatment of specific metabolic disorders are described elsewhere (See hyperkalemia, metabolic acidosis etc.).

Avoid nephrotoxic drugs: NSAIDs, aminoglycosides, ACEI. Aminoglycoside antibiotics can be used if essential, but dosage and frequency of administration should be adjusted for loss of excretory renal capacity. As a general principle, loading doses should be as normal, but maintenance doses need to be smaller and/or less frequent.

If the cause of ARF is acute interstitial nephritis, any offending medication or therapy must be discontinued. Steroids have been used (with no controlled trials) either as pulse IV methylprednisolone 500–1000 mg/d for 3–4 days or short courses of prednisolone 60 mg od PO for 2 weeks with a rapid taper (See Interstitial nephritis).

Glomerulonephritis (GN) may be isolated or part of a systemic disease. Cellular casts and/or large numbers of dysmorphic red blood cells in the urinary sediment suggest GN. Renal biopsy is required to establish the nature of the glomerular lesion (see "Glomerulonephritis").

Treatment of post renal ARF is relief of obstruction and the prognosis depends upon the cause of the obstruction and the duration of impaired urinary drainage. Bladder outflow obstruction can be relieved by urethral or suprapubic bladder catheterization, obstruction higher up the urinary tract may require percutaneous nephrostomy and/or ureteric stents.

Proper nutrition and diet high in protein and calories must be assured, orally if possible. Gastric or jejunal feeding tube or TPN may be required.

As for other patients requiring Intensive care, consider gastric protection with proton pump inhibitor omeprazole 10-40 mg daily PO or H2 antagonist ranitidine 150 mg bd PO, or 50 mg bd IM or 50 mg diluted in 20 ml 5% Glucose or 0.9% saline IV slowly over 2 minutes. These may reduce the risk of gastrointestinal hemorrhage.

ADULT POLYCYSTIC KIDNEY DISEASE (APCKD)

Cyst drainage

Direct reduction of cyst size by percutaneous aspiration, aspiration with sclerosis, or surgical drainage has been effectively used to relieve severe or refractory pain; there is, however, no evidence that these measures improve renal function or delay the rate of disease progression.

Hypertension in APCKD patient

Patients with hypertension and APCKD generally respond well to ACE inhibitors. In addition to lowering systemic pressures, ACE inhibitor therapy also can reverse left ventricular hypertrophy. The aim of antihypertensive therapy should be to lower the blood pressure to 130-140/80-85 mm Hg, similar to that in patients with essential hypertension.

Pain in APCKD

NSAIDs (nonselective inhibitors of both COX-1 and COX-2 and selective COX-2 inhibitors) could be given for 3-5 days with good hydration, but this is controversial. Opiate analgaesia may be required: start with mildest. Remember that opiate drugs and their metabolites accumulate in patients with impaired excretory renal function: this is a particular problem with pethidine, and to a lesser extent with codeine. Hydromorphone is a useful analgaesic in patients with renal impairment.

Protein restriction

There are conflicting findings on the efficacy of a low protein diet (0.6 to 0.7 g/kg per day). At present, we do not recommend restriction of protein intake below 1 to 1.1 g/kg per day in patients with APCKD given the limited evidence of benefit.

Renal replacement therapy

Patients with APCKD who progress to end-stage renal disease require renal replacement therapy. In general, such patients have equivalent or perhaps better overall outcomes with any renal replacement therapy compared to non-APCKD patients. Patients are most commonly treated with hemodialysis or undergo renal transplantation. Peritoneal dialysis is less commonly performed. This is due in part to the reduced intraabdominal space available for effective peritoneal exchange in the presence of massively enlarged kidneys. Nevertheless, some centres have found that peritoneal dialysis is well tolerated and results in no specific difficulties in the patient with APCKD requiring renal replacement therapy. Some patients require pretransplant native nephrectomy to better accommodate the graft.

Urinary Tract Infection in APCKD

Patients with pyuria and positive urine cultures should be treated according to the result of antibiotic sensitivity testing. The most frequently used oral drugs are amoxicillin (250 or 500 mg tds PO); trimethoprim 200 mg bd PO (causes an artefactual rise in plasma creatinine due to inhibition of tubular secretion of creatinine); ciprofloxacin 250 or 500 mg bd PO. If parenteral antibiotic therapy is indicated an alternative is gentamicin single dose 180 mg od IM/IV over 3 min, followed by maintenance dose adjusted according to renal function and regular measurement of gentamicin levels in blood. Treatment duration 10–14 days (see Urinary tract infections).

In complicated urinary tract infection (infected cyst) use antibiotics that penetrate cyst such as quinolones (ciprofloxacin 500 mg bd PO or 400 mg bd IV), trimethoprim (200 mg bd PO), co-trimoxazole (960 mg bd PO) or chloramphenicol 250 mg qds PO or 50 mg/kg/d IV). Chloramphenicol is reserved for treatment of life-threatening conditions.

If infection is due to streptococci or staphylococci use Vancomycin 1 g/d slow IV over 100 min, trough blood level should not be > 10 mg/dl; or Erythromycin 250 – 500 mg qds PO or 25 – 50 mg/kg/d either by continuous infusion or in divided doses every 6 h.

If infection is due to anaerobic microorganisms use Metronidazole 500 mg tds PO or in severe infection 500 mg tds IV.

Cyst infection needs treatment for at least 4–6 weeks. Surgical drainage is indicated if perinephric abscess develops.

Nephrectomy is indicated in patients with severe infection refractory to antibiotic therapy and also in some patients who will undergo renal transplantation to minimize recidivant infection during immunosuppressive therapy.

ANALGAESICS

Aspirin, enteric-coated aspirin, buffered aspirin: 75-300 mg up to 4 times/day.

In addition, low dose aspirin is often used for vascular protection (75 mg daily is convenient because of the availability of this tablet size as paediatric aspirin; even lower doses may be equally effective).

Avoid all NSAIDs when there is an increased risk of gastro-intestinal bleeding. In mild renal impairment use the lowest effective dose and monitor renal function, sodium and water retention. If used, the dosage is as follows:

Ibuprofen 1.2–2.4 g/day in 3-4 divided doses

Indomethacin 50 – 200 mg/day in 3-4 divided doses

Diclofenac (Voltarol) 75–120 mg/day in 3-4 divided doses

Others:

Paracetamol (acetaminophen) 1 g every 4-6 hours, max. 4 g daily
Co-dydramol 1-2 tablets every 4-6 hours, max. 8 tablets daily
Co-proxamol 2 tablets 3-4 times daily, max. 8 tablets daily
Co-codamol 30/500 1-2 tablets every 4 hours, max. 8 tablets daily
Codeine and its metabolites may accumulate in renal failure, so be aware of insidious onset of respiratory depression or other opiate adverse effects.
Tramadol 50 mg–100 mg, max 400 mg daily PO; 50 mg by IM or IV injection
Pethidine may accumulate in renal failure, therefore morphine is preferable. Morphine sulphate SC/IM injections 10 mg every 4 hours. For IV injection use ½ of IM dose.
Morphine oral solutions: eg Oramorph 10 mg/5 ml. Morphine tablets: eg Sevredol tbl 10 mg every 4 hours.
Hydromorphone (Palladone) is particularly useful in patients with renal disease, including those on dialysis. Capsule sizes are 1.3 mg or 2.6 mg and the drug must be given at 4 hourly intervals. Dose can be escalated to achieve pain control.
Fentanyl patches (self-adhesive patches delivering transcutaneous drug) provide a convenient form of administration of continuous potent analgaesic. Patches are available in a range of doses and typically last for 72 hours.

ANAPHYLACTIC SHOCK

Adrenaline (epinephrine) 1:1000, 0.3-0.5 ml IM is preferred route since absorption more reliable than via SC route. IV administration of adrenaline (epinephrine) 0.5–1 mL of 1:10,000 solution is reserved for dire emergencies. Adrenaline injection can be repeated every 5-10 minutes until recovered (according to pulse, BP, respiratory function).
Chlorpheniramine maleate (Piriton) 10 mg IM/IV
Hydrocortisone 200 mg IV. Dose can be repeated after 6 h.
Oxygen at 100% 12 L/hour
If patient is hypotensive/hypovolemic (BP<90 mm Hg) give IV infusion of 500 ml 0.9% saline or 500 ml colloid (eg Haemaccel) over 15 min.

ANTICOAGULATION

Many patients with renal disease are taking aspirin or anticoagulants and the general principles are similar to those in non-renal patients. Low molecular weight heparins should be used with caution in patients with impaired renal function.

Anticardiolipin antibodies

Patients with anticardiolipin antibodies who have a history of venous or arterial thrombosis should be anticoagulated for at least 12 months and preferably for life and/or the duration of antibody positivity.

Anticoagulation regimen before surgery

Risks associated with temporary cessation of anticoagulation depend upon the original reason for anticoagulation: risks are highest for patients with prosthetic heart valves in whom anticoagulation should be maintained, even at lower intensity, if possible. By contrast, anticoagulation for reasons associated with haemodialysis access patency can usually be temporarily interrupted without difficulty.

Where reversal of anticoagulation is deemed essential: if INR is 2-3, discontinue warfarin 4 days before surgery. Aim for INR less than 1.5 on the day of surgery. If one day before operation INR is >1.8 give 1 mg vitamin K SC and check INR 24 hours later. If INR is still high on the day of operation, give 3 units of fresh frozen plasma (FFP), it will have an effect that may last for 10 hours.

If patient is on IV heparin: stop heparin six hours before surgery. Delay heparin injections/infusions for 12 hours after surgery.

If patient was on warfarin, re-start warfarin as soon as possible after surgery. Administration of vitamin K renders patients more difficult to adequately re-anticoagulate so should be avoided if possible.

Heparin infusion

Check PT and APTT. Initiate therapy with 5000 u heparin IV over 5 minutes followed by heparin 1000 u/hr. Add 25,000 u heparin to 50 ml isotonic saline to have heparin 500 u/ml in a syringe pump. Start at 1000 units per hour (2 ml/h).

Check APTT 6 hours after starting heparin infusion or 6 hours after adjusting the dose. Aim for APTT ratio 1.8-2.5. Adjust the dose as follows:

APTT ratio	Change rate u/h by
5.1–7	− 500
4.1–5	− 300
3.1–4	− 100
2.6–3	− 50
1.5–2.5	0
1.2–1.4	+ 200
< 1.2	+ 400

− Means reduce the dose by…
+ Means increase the dose by….

Start warfarin the same day. Heparin therapy is overlapped with warfarin for a minimum of 5 days; heparin should be discontinued on 4th or 5th day provided that the INR is in therapeutic range (eg for venous thromboembolism INR 2.0-3.0).

Prophylactic anticoagulation

Routine prophylaxis for surgical/medical patients: Unfractionated **heparin** SC 5000 u every 12 hours for 7 days or until patient is ambulant.

Low molecular weight heparins are as effective and safe as unfractionated heparin in the prevention of venous thromboembolism. The standard prophylactic regimen does not require monitoring. In severe renal impairment, the risk of bleeding during heparin treatment is increased and low molecular weight heparins are best avoided.

Enoxaparin (Clexane) subcutaneous injections for prophylaxis of DVT especially in *surgical patients*:

moderate risk: 20 mg (2000 units) approx. 2 hours before surgery then 20 mg (2000 units) every 24 hours for 7-10 days

high risk: 40 mg (4000 units) 12 hours before surgery then 40 mg (4000 units) every 24 hours for 7-10 days.

Prophylaxis of DVT in medical patients: 40 mg (4000 units) every 24 hours for at least 6 days until patient ambulant (max.14 days).

Deltaparin sodium (Fragmin) subcutaneous injections for *prophylaxis of DVT*:

> moderate risk: 2500 units 1-2 hours before surgery, then 2500 units every 24 hours for 5-7 days
>
> high risk: 2500 units 1-2 hours before surgery; then 2500 units twice daily (or 5000 units once daily).

Compression stockings and ambulation are basic measures that complement the medication.

Pulmonary embolism (PE) and deep vein thrombosis (DVT)

In addition to specific procedures: oxygen 100% (unless COPD) and pain relief (morphine 10 mg IV), anticoagulate with standard unfractionated heparin (see above) followed by warfarin.

Patients with a single episode of DVT or PE should receive warfarin for 6 months; those with recurrent thrombosis or embolism or atrial fibrillation may require prolonged therapy and in those with prosthetic heart valves or other intravascular device, lifelong therapy is normally indicated.

Warfarin dosage

Check baseline INR before starting warfarin therapy. If normal, a suggested initiation regimen is to give 10 mg warfarin daily for two consecutive days. Commence warfarin on day 0 (and give subsequent daily doses) at 17.00 h.

Check INR the following morning and adjust the doses of warfarin:

Day	INR	Dose (mg)	Maintenance (mg)
1	<1.4	10	
2	<1.8	10	
3	<2	10	6
	2	5	5.5
	2.5	4	4.5
	2.9	3	4
	3.3	2	3.5
	3.6	0.5	3
	4.1	0	*

* Miss dose, and give the following day 1 mg; if INR >4.5 miss two doses

The daily dose of warfarin should be adjusted according to the target INR:

Condition	INR
Prevention of DVT	2–3
Treatment of DVT or PE	2–3
AF	2–3
Acute MI	3–4.5
Mechanical prosthetic heart valve	3–4.9

The dose may be altered according to clinical circumstances.

Therapy for idiopathic venous thromboembolism typically includes a 5-to-10-day course of heparin followed by 3 to 12 months of oral anticoagulation therapy with full dose warfarin, with adjustment of dose to achieve an international normalized ratio (INR) between 2.0 and 3.0.

Reversal of anticoagulation is done in patients on warfarin who are undergoing surgical procedures. If INR>1.5 give 2 units of FFP (600 mL) IV over 1 hour plus vit K 1 mg IV (if INR>3 vit K 2 mg IV stat).

ANTIPHOSPHOLIPID ANTIBODY SYNDROME (APS)

Prophylaxis of recurrent arterial/venous thrombo-embolic events includes the following:

Prophylaxis of DVT

Aspirin + heparin or warfarin.
Aspirin 75–150 mg once a day
Target INR of 2.5–3.5 for all patients with APS treated with oral anticoagulants.
Most patients with definite APS and previous thrombosis should be treated to a target INR of 3.5. The exception could be individuals with only venous events and those at high risk of bleeding, who could be considered for lower intensities of anticoagulation.
Anticoagulate with warfarin indefinitely.
Warfarin is teratogenic and it should not be used in pregnant women.
Do not give anticoagulation if platelet count is less than $50 \times 10^9/l$.

Pregnancy in association with antiphospholipid antibodies

Warfarin is teratogenic! Heparin plus low dose aspirin is more effective than aspirin alone for achieving live birth among women with antiphospholipid antibodies.

Women with history of pregnancy loss, history of thrombotic events or high titre of IgG antiphospholipid antibodies may be treated with 5000 u of unfractionated heparin twice daily. Standard heparin may be substituted for low molecular weight heparin in the treatment of pregnant women with antiphospholipid antibody syndrome:

Deltaparin 5000 – 10000 u od SC + aspirin 75–100 mg od PO.

ASCITES

Salt restriction.
Frusemide 40–120 mg/24 hours + Spironolactone 100 mg/24 hours. Repeated large–volume paracentesis (4–6 litres) with albumin infusion. Six to 8 g of albumin/litre of ascitic fluid removed is administered intravenously during or after the procedure to prevent relative hypovolemia, which usually occurs 3–6 hours later.

ATRIAL FIBRILLATION (AF)

AF is common in patients with renal disease. Short episodes may occur in haemodialysis patients due to volume shifts. Sustained or paroxysmal AF can be managed similarly to non–renal patients with the exception that digoxin is renally excreted and the maintenance dose and frequency must be reduced.

In a patient who presents with AF and a rapid ventricular response rate, there needs to be an urgent assessment for underlying causes such as heart failure, pulmonary problems, hypertension, or hyperthyroidism. Treatment of these conditions may result in reversion to sinus rhythm.

Two standard approaches to converting AF to sinus rhythm are synchronized electrical DC cardioversion and pharmacological cardioversion.

DC cardioversion is indicated in patients who are haemodynamically unstable. The role for cardioversion depends upon the duration of the arrhythmia as well as the presence of a reversible aetiological factor.

If the duration of the arrhythmia is 48 hours or less and there are no associated cardiac abnormalities (particularly mitral valve disease or significant left ventricular enlargement due to a cardiomyopathy), there is a low risk of systemic embolization and electrical or pharmacological cardioversion can be attempted after systemic heparinization. Anticoagulation is indicated for three to four weeks after cardioversion.

Patients who have been in AF for more than 48 hours should receive three to four weeks of warfarin prior to and after cardioversion with a target INR of 2.5 (range 2.0 to 3.0).

Medical control of AF and fast ventricular rate can be achieved with amiodarone, digoxin, calcium channel blocker, beta–blocker.

Amiodarone (300 mg in 5% dextrose IV over 20–120 minutes followed by 900 mg in 500 ml 5% dextrose over 24 hours, concomitantly oral 200 mg tds for week one, 200 mg bd for week two and maintenance 200 mg od) may be preferred in patients with a reduced left ventricular ejection fraction.

Digoxin is usually the preferred drug in patients with AF due to heart failure. Digoxin can also be used in patients who cannot take or who respond inadequately to beta–blockers or calcium channel blockers. The dose of digoxin: initiate with two doses of 0.5 mg PO 12 hours apart, followed by 0.25 mg 12 hourly for 2 days. Maintenance dose of digoxin is 0.0625–0.125 mg/day (reduce dose and/or frequency of administration in renal impairment).

In most other situations, a beta blocker or calcium channel blocker is preferred since, in the absence of heart failure, digoxin is less effective for rate control than beta blockers and calcium channel blockers, is less likely to control the ventricular rate during exercise (when vagal tone is low and sympathetic tone is high), has little or no ability to terminate the arrhythmia, and often does not slow the heart rate with recurrent AF.

Beta blockers (sotalol 40–80–160 mg 12 hourly or atenolol 50 mg od) and non-dihydropyridine calcium channel blockers (verapamil 40–120 mg bd PO or diltiazem 60 mg tds or diltiazem SR 60–90–120 mg bd PO) are also effective if heart failure or hypotension is due to the rapid arrhythmia. NB Diltiazem interacts with calcineurin inhibitors (cyclosporin and tacrolimus) to cause raised cyclosporin/tacrolimus blood levels: in renal transplant recipients or other patients taking these drugs caution is required, plus increased frequency of measurement of blood levels.

Maintenance anticoagulation with warfarin is superior to aspirin. If aspirin is given the dose should be 75–300 mg/day PO.

BACTERIAL ENDOCARDITIS

Take multiple blood cultures before initiating antibiotic therapy if possible. "Blind" therapy: benzyl penicillin 1.2 g four hourly IV + gentamicin for 2 weeks followed by amoxicillin 1 g TDS for 2 weeks. Specific therapy according to the result of blood cultures. Gentamicin dose should be adjusted according to renal function and blood levels should be closely monitored. Renal toxicity can occur even if recommended therapeutic levels are not exceeded, especially if there is co-administration of loop diuretics.

BLADDER CATHETERIZATION (antibiotic prophylaxis)

Just before the intervention start prophylaxis with either: ciprofloxacin 250 mg bd PO for two days or co-trimoxazole (Septrin) 960 mg bd PO for two days.

BODY SURFACE AREA (BSA)

Appropriate dosage of some drugs used in patients with renal disease is calculated on the basis of body surface area
Body surface area = square root of [height (cm) X weight (kg)/3600]
Nowadays one can use medical calculators or internet site to simplify the calculation of BSA.

BOWEL PREPARATION IN RENAL PATIENTS

Problems with fluid load and risk of severe hyperphosphataemia make "conventional" bowel preparations, eg for colonoscopy, potentially hazardous in patients with renal disease, especially those on dialysis. Picolax (sodium picosulfate with magnesium citrate) is usually effective. One sachet (10 mg), reconstituted in a cup of approximately 150 ml of water, is given 24 hours before procedure and a further sachet 6–8 hours later. Patients on a fluid restriction may need reassessment to compensate for fluid losses during Picolax treatment.

BRADYCARDIA

Stop beta-blockers.
Give atropine 500 µg IV (maximum 3 mg).
The patient may need transvenous pacing if bradycardia is persistent. In an emergency, IV injection of glucagon (50–150 micrograms/kg in 5% glucose) may be lifesaving. Precautions should be taken to protect the airway in case of vomiting.

CANDIDIASIS

Local treatment: nystatin 100,000 u/ml, 1 ml four times/day after food for 7 days, or continue therapy for 48 hours after lesions have resolved; amphotericin B lozenges 4–6 times/d. Amphotericin is preferable because it takes 30 min or so to suck the lozenges. Nystatin suspension can be used as a wash solution for false teeth.

For invasive or systemic candida infection use fluconazole as the least toxic but effective anti-fungal drug.

Mucosal candidiasis: fluconazole 50 mg/day for 14 days.

Oropharyngeal candidiasis: fluconazole day one 200 mg; then 100 mg/day for at least 14 days.

Oesophageal candidiasis: fluconazole day 200 mg on day 1; then 100 mg/day for a minimum of 21 days and for at least 14 days following resolution of symptoms.

Systemic candidiasis: fluconazole 6 mg/kg/d on first day then 3–6 mg/kg/d. For 70 kg patient this would be 400 mg PO or IV day 1, then 200 mg/daily PO or IV, continue treatment according to the response for at least 28 days.

NB Fluconazole interacts with calcineurin inhibitors (cyclosporin and tacrolimus) to cause raised cyclosporin/tacrolimus blood levels: in renal transplant recipients or other patients taking these drugs caution is required, plus increased frequency of measurement of blood levels.

Amphotericin B is the standard therapy for the treatment of severe, invasive or life-threatening systemic fungal infections. Method of administration: prepare IV infusion by dissolving amphotericin B in 5% dextrose to a final concentration 0.1 mg/mL. Give a test dose of 1 mg (10 mL of initial infusion) over 20–30 minutes, then 0.25 – 0.5 – 1.0 mg/kg (depending on the severity of infection) IV infusion over 4 to 6 hours.

The duration of therapy depends on many variables, but generally high risk patients should be treated for 10 – 14 days after disappearance of symptoms and after the last positive fungal blood culture.

Lipid (liposomal) formulations of amphotericin B are more effective and less toxic (but more expensive). Dose: Abelcet (Wyeth) 5 mg/ml, give as IV infusion, initial test dose 1 mg over 15 minutes, then 5 mg/kg daily for at least 14 days. AmBisome (NeXStar) initial dose 1 mg over 10 minutes then 1 mg/kg daily as a single dose increased gradually if necessary to 3 mg/kg daily as a single dose.

Flucytosine could be used as an additional anti-fungal agent in combination with either amphotericin B or fluconazole for treatment of refractory infections. The dose of flucytosine is 25–50 mg/kg qds IV for up to 7 days.

Caspofungin is a new antifungal drug, with fungicidal activity (against Aspergillus and most Candida species). Administer as a single daily dose of either 50 or 70 mg in 200 ml 0.9% saline IV over 1-h period followed by an infusion of saline 200 ml over the next hour.

CAPD (CONTINUOUS AMBULATORY PERITONEAL DIALYSIS)

Antibiotic prophylaxis before PD catheter insertion (Tenckhoff catheter is most commonly used, this name tends to be used generically to mean any PD catheter)

Vancomycin 1 g IV 12 h before the procedure and
Cephalozin 0.5–1 g 3 h before the procedure

Bloody Peritoneal Dialysis (PD) fluid

Hemorrhage may be benign (retrograde menstruation, minor trauma) and will need treatment if associated with drainage problems (add heparin 500 u to each bag of CAPD fluid). More serious causes of bloody PD fluids are ruptured vessels and may require surgical exploration.

CAPD solutions

Dianeal: basic glucose/lactate based solution available in three different strengths of glucose: 1.36% (isotonic), 2.27% or 3.86%, getting more hypertonic as the % increases. Each of the three strengths are available in different volumes; the volumes frequently used are 0.5, 1, 1.5, 2, 2.5 and 3 litres.

Nutrineal: 1.1% amino acid solution. Isotonic in terms of its ultrafiltration ability. Used to increase serum albumin levels. A patient can have only one bag (2 L) per 24 hours. Patient must be adequately dialyzed before you start it as the serum urea will go up with the protein absorption. Also used for patients with diabetes mellitus to replace 1 bag a day to reduce sugar calorie load. Better biocompatibility than glucose fluid (Dianeal).

Extraneal: synonym Icodextrin 7.5%. This solution is used for sustained ultrafiltration to control fluid balance. Needs long dwell in usually 8–10 hours, but 6 hours as absolute minimum. Good for "high transporters" who retain fluid badly on long dwells otherwise. Good for patients with diabetes mellitus as can not absorb any glucose load since it is a glucose polymer and the molecule is too big to go through the membrane. If a patient is on insulin and already on CAPD and then a bag is swapped to Extraneal, you have to reduce the insulin that covers that dwell as there is then no glucose absorption where there was before. Only one bag per 24 hours (get maltose build up as a breakdown product).

Physioneal: bicarbonate based fluid in same strengths as Dianeal. Better biocompatibility as no GDP (glucose degradation products) from heat sterilizing as the bag is in 2 compartments until about to be run in to the patient. Also referred as AGE's (advanced glycosylation end products) which do the damage to the peritoneal membrane long term.

Catheter blockage or poor drainage of CAPD fluid

Check X – ray plain film of the abdomen to see whether the catheter is malpositioned.

If catheter is flipped in upper abdominal quadrants administer laxatives: senna 2–4 tbl od PO usually at night or lactulose 15 ml od PO. If the catheter does not flip to lower abdominal quadrant give more potent laxative eg sodium picosulfate one sachet of 10 mg od PO. Finally, if all these measures are without effect, and if there is an expertise - try various guide wire techniques. If all of these procedures fail, there may be a need for surgical repositioning, laparoscopic if possible.

If the blockage is due to fibrin use urokinase either 25,000 U in 2 ml saline, leave in the catheter for 2–4 hours or make up to 50 ml with isotonic saline and infuse into catheter via a pump at 2 ml/min for 24 h. Alternative is heparin 5,000 u plus urokinase 5,000 u made up to 50 ml with isotonic saline.

Colonoscopy in CAPD patient

Drain the dialysate before the procedure. After the procedure inject gentamicin into the bag and leave for 6 hours, the dose of gentamicin is dependent on the body weight (see below).

Contamination protocol for peritoneal dialysis

(Split patient line or Tenckhoff; titanium connector pulled out or disconnected; hole in PD fluid bag or lines; touch contamination followed by PD fluid flow)

Vancomycin 500 mg, distilled water for injection 10 ml, 10 ml syringe, green or orange needle. Connect 10 ml syringe and green needle. Draw up 10 ml of distilled water and add to vancomycin powder. Shake gently to mix and withdraw all 10 ml into the same syringe. Change to orange needle. Inject into new PD bag. Mix well. Drain in dialysis fluid and leave for 6 hours. Continue dialysis as normal.

The other alternative is gentamicin. Gentamicin dose dependent on the weight of patient:

Patient weight (kg)	dose of gentamicin (mg)
20–40	40
41–60	60
61–100	80
101 or more	120

You need: vials of gentamicin; 5 ml syringe; green and orange needle. Connect 5 ml syringe and green needle. Draw up appropriate dose into syringe. Change to orange needle. Inject into a new PD bag. Mix well. Drain in dialysis fluid and leave for at least 6 hours. Continue dialysis as normal.

Cefazolin 1 g IP can be used to avoid vancomycin and gentamicin.

Exit site infection

Take swab for culture and sensitivity testing prior to starting antibiotics. Flucloxacillin 500 mg qds PO for 2 weeks, followed by 250 mg qds PO for 1 week, and if refractory Staphylococcus aureus isolated add Rifampicin 450 mg od PO for the first 2 weeks.

If the patient is penicillin allergic:
Erythromycin 500 mg qds PO for 2 weeks followed by 250 mg qds PO, for 1 week + Fucidin 500 mg tds for the first two weeks. Fucidin is often poorly tolerated.

If infection is due to Gram negative bacteria:
Ciprofloxacin 500 mg bd PO or 400 mg bd IV for 3–4 weeks.

Recurrent or refractory infections with Staphylococcus aureus: Rifampicin 300 mg bd PO, duration of treatment 12 weeks. Consider catheter removal.

Vancomycin (for gram-positive microorganisms) and gentamicin (for gram-negative microorganism) are still widely used in the treatment of exit site infections (for the doses see Peritonitis below)

Local mupirocin (Bactroban) treatment during routine exit site care in all patients on PD and specially in patients who are known staphylococcus aureus carriers, who have had an exit site infection, tunnel infection or peritonitis with staphylococcus aureus.
The use of mupirocin should be continued indefinitely.

Exit site infections are often persistent and may only be cured by removal of catheter. This is especially true if a tunnel infection develops.

Intra-peritoneal insulin

Patients with diabetes mellitus can administer insulin via the intra-peritoneal route to minimise number of subcutaneous injections. Short-acting soluble insulin should be used (eg Actrapid). PD fluids are usually dextrose-based and patients will require an increased insulin dosage compared to pre-PD. Total daily insulin dose via the intra-peritoneal route will probably need to be 25–30% higher than previous total daily subcutaneous dose but to err on the side of safety and avoid hypoglycaemia, it is often best to start by administering same total daily dose by IP route (see below), monitor blood sugar before each exchange and adjust accordingly. Patient may need to be admitted to hospital for close observation during this period. For overnight PD bag, add 12 units of soluble insulin. For daytime bags, divide remainder of total daily dose (ie total minus 12) by number of bags (usually 3) and administer equal insulin doses in each bag. Hypertonic bags require a larger dose of insulin.

Pain on drainage

Instill in the abdominal cavity via PD catheter and prior to commencing daily exchanges 5 ml of 8.4% sodium bicarbonate.

If bicarbonate does not help, and very rarely, use 2 ml 2% lignocaine.

Physioneal (if it is available) may also help in reducing the pain on drainage.

Peritonitis

Drain PD bag and send to laboratory for microscopy, culture and sensitivity testing.
Patients with severe abdominal pain should have 3 rapid lavages to ease pain, but this should not be continued since lavaging reduces peritoneal defence.
Initial therapy: Vancomycin IP (if body weight>90 kg = 2.5 g; 70–90 kg = 2 g; 40–70 kg = 1.5 g <40 kg = 1 g). Drain in over 60–90 min and leave to dwell for 6 hours.
From day 0 also ciprofloxacin 500 mg bd until culture and antibiotic sensitivities are available (usually 48 hours). Peritonitis is associated with increased generation of fibrin, which may occlude catheter, therefore when CAPD fluid is cloudy heparin 1000 U IP should be added to each bag in all subsequent bags whilst cloudy.

Protocol based on the use of first generation of cephalosporin such as cefazolin or cephalothin in combination with ceftazidime is recommended with patients with residual renal function:

Gram-positive: Cefazolin 15 mg/kg od (single dose) IP initially for 24–48 h, if MRSA isolated substitute vancomycin for cephazolin (dose see below). It is usual practice to use an additional antibiotic to cover gram-negative microorganisms (Ceftazidime 1 g od IP).

The loading dose of antibiotics is best administered in 1 L bag of PD fluid.

Sample prescription:

Infuse 1 l of 1.5% dextrose dialysis solution containing:

1 g Cefazolin
0.5 g ceftazidime
1000 u heparin

Dwell for 3 h.

In patients who are septic administer antibiotics IV instead of IP (Cefazolin 1 g od IV and ceftazidime 1 g od IV).

Maintenance dosage: continue regular CAPD schedule, add 125 mg/L ceftazidime, 125 mg/L Cefazolin and 1000 u heparin to each bag.

APD patient may be temporarily converted to CAPD during the treatment of peritonitis.

Protocol based on aminoglycosides in patients without residual renal function:

Gram positive organism isolated: stop ciprofloxacin. Administer vancomycin on day 7, the same dose as on day 0. If there is no improvement in the patient after 3–4 days prior to sensitivities becoming available, then it may be appropriate to add rifampicin 600 mg/day for gram-positive infections, particularly Staphylococcus aureus. In severe cases of Staphylococcus aureus peritonitis, 3 weeks therapy is appropriate and catheter removal may occasionally be necessary.

Gram negative microorganism isolated: stop vancomycin.
Continue ciprofloxacin for 14 days or modify as appropriate to sensitivities when received or to clinical response.

If resistant gram-negative microorganisms were isolated, discontinue ciprofloxacin and inject gentamicin 8 mg/l into each bag (i.e. 16 mg/two litre PD solution).

Single gram-negative infections that are not responding to ciprofloxacin should be managed with gentamicin, ceftazidime

(ceftazidime 1 g bd IV) or aztreonam according to sensitivities. Mixed infections suggest bowel pathology (see below).

Pseudomonas aeruginosa infections should probably be treated for a total 3 weeks with 2 separate drugs, i.e. gentamicin and ceftazidime or gentamicin and aztreonam. Catheter removal is often necessary.

If there has been no improvement in clinical condition after a few days, or if the patient is septic, then hospital admission is often appropriate and clinical assessment to exclude a bowel perforation is warranted. Failure to improve is often an indication for catheter removal. This is particularly likely in infections with Pseudomonas, resistant Staphylococci or fungi.

Oral ciprofloxacin is unlikely to be adequate therapy for multiple gram-negative organisms (i.e. suspected bowel leak). These patients will require inpatient care with metronidazole, gentamicin and fluconazole in combination with surgical assessment.

Fungal peritonitis: if fungi are isolated as a cause of peritonitis, catheter removal will often prove necessary. If the patient is not severely unwell try for a few days to salvage the catheter using fluconazole 200 mg od PO plus flucytosine 0.5–1 g od by IV infusion over 20–40 minutes. An alternative is liposomal amphotericin B (see below).

In most cases the catheter should be removed the same day. A central line is inserted for haemodialysis and a second line for IV amphotericin that is administered as follows:

Day 1: 0.25 mg/kg in 250 ml 5% dextrose over 6 hours
Day 2: 0.5 mg/kg in 250 ml 5% dextrose over 6 hours
Day 3: 0.75 mg/kg in 250 ml 5% dextrose over 6 hours.

In addition to catheter removal the PO or IV administration of antifungal drugs especially flucytosine reduce incidence of peritoneal adhesions.

Placement of a new catheter should not be attempted for at least 8 weeks following treatment and at least 1 week after all clinical evidence of peritonitis has subsided.

No bacterial growth: if there is no growth by day 3 or 4 then stop ciprofloxacin unless there have been previous episodes of gram negative peritonitis and continue as per gram-positive microorganisms. The outcome of no growth peritonitis is usually favorable; however patient should be monitored carefully for possible bowel perforation or fungal peritonitis.

Refractory peritonitis of any etiology: if for any reason the episode of peritonitis does not clear within 3–4 days of appropriate antibiotics, it may be necessary to remove the catheter as a matter of urgency.

Heparin: add heparin 500–1000 u per L of dialysis solution until symptoms and signs of peritonitis have resolved and until fibrinous clots are no longer visible.

The use of hypertonic glucose solutions is common in the early stages of peritonitis, and adjustments in prescriptions are usually required until the inflammatory process has completely abated.

Persistent tunnel infection

Remove the catheter and insert new catheter after 4 weeks.

CARPAL TUNNEL SYNDROME

Patients on dialysis usually do not respond to conservative therapy and we go to surgery straight away.

Conservative therapies that may be tried are:
- Nocturnal splints
- Simple analgaesics
- NSAIDs or corticosteroids for acute pain relief. Oral prednisolone 20 mg daily for 7 days followed by 10 mg daily for another 7 days.
- Steroid injections into carpal tunnel (20–40 mg Methylprednisolone).
- Ultrasound therapy

CELLULITIS

Cellulitis is common in patients with oedema: in nephrotic syndrome there is added susceptibility to infection since hypogammaglobulinaemia is often associated.
Initial antibiotic therapy is usually empirical, so antimicrobial coverage should include agents that are effective against beta-hemolytic streptococci and staphylococcus aureus:

- cefazolin 1 to 2 g tds IV
- phenoxymethylpenicillin (Penicillin V) 500 mg qds + flucloxacillin 500 mg qds for two weeks; or
- cefuroxime 500 mg bd PO; or
- cephalexin 500 mg qds PO.
- combination of trimethoprim (200 mg bd pO) and Rifampicin 300 mg bd-qds PO (for more severe staphylococcal infections)

In more severe cellulitis a later generation cephalosporin such as ceftriaxone 2 g IM or IV provides coverage for beta-hemolytic streptococci and staphylococcus aureus.

Patients allergic to penicillin may receive clindamycin 600 mg tds IV to treat beta-hemolytic streptococci and staphylococcus aureus.

Vancomycin can also be used to treat proven or strongly suspected gram-positive infections or MRSA (methicillin resistant staphylococcus aureus) carriers; the dose is 1 g bd if renal function is normal. In renal insufficiency 1 g of vancomycin can be given and subsequent doses only after checking pre-dose (trough) level that should be <10 mg/l.

Fluoroquinolones can be used if gram-negative pathogens are suspected or proven (ciprofloxacin 400 mg bd IV or 500 mg bd PO).

CEREBRAL OEDEMA

Urgent CT scan and neurosurgical opinion. Patients on HD have an increased risk of subdural haematoma. Dexamethasone 10 mg IV stat, then 4 mg IV/IM every 6 hours while symptoms persist then taper and switch to oral.

CHOLESTEROL CRYSTAL ATHEROEMBOLIC RENAL DISEASE (synonyms cholesterol embolism, athero-embolism)

Although many different agents have been evaluated such as steroids and statins, there is no currently effective medical therapy.

Withdrawal of anticoagulants may stop further dislodgement of cholesterol crystals. Lower the blood pressure in hypertensive patients.

Heparin-free dialysis could also reduce or stop further cholesterol crystal embolism.

To prevent cholesterol crystal embolism, the brachial instead of femoral approach in heart or renal angiography could be used, as there are usually many more atherosclerotic plaques in the abdominal aorta.

CHRONIC RENAL INSUFFICIENCY (CRI)

Dialysis if conservative treatment ineffective, failing to control symptoms, and/or when GFR <5 ml/min, assuming that patient wishes to receive dialysis after appropriate education and counselling. Dialysis outcomes are improved if period of carefeul planning is available: during this time access for dialysis can be prepared (fistula, Tenckhoff catheter, permcath dual lumen IV line).

Treat reversible contributors: infection, obstruction, electrolyte imbalance, heart failure, hypertension, stop or minimise nephrotoxic drugs (NSAIDs, aminoglycosides). Do not use ACEI or AIIRA in patients with bilateral renal artery stenosis, but in other causes of renal insufficiency these drugs have useful effects, can slow down the progression to renal failure and also reduce proteinuria in proteinuric patients. ACEI and AIIRA cause hyperkalaemia: monitor serum potassium concentration.

Anaemia of CRI

Target Haemoglobin (Hb) 11–12 g/L, haematocrit 33–36%.
Avoid blood transfusion, but give leukocyte-depleted blood if the patient is symptomatic of anaemia and Hb <7 g/l.

Iron utilisation is ineffective in CRI, so "functional" iron deficiency may exist in the face of apparently adequate iron stores. Remember also that plasma ferritin is an acute phase reactant and may be artefactually elevated during intercurrent illness especially infections. Correct iron deficit first. Indications for iron supplement: ferritin <100ug/l (optimum 200ug/l–500ug/l); transferrin saturation <20%, % hypochromic red blood cells >10%.

Oral iron: Ferrous sulphate 200 mg tds intitially. Oral iron may have poor absorption, side effects, and most important – oral iron supplements are often ineffective in treating iron deficiency in patients on chronic haemodialysis. Oral iron should not be taken at the same time as phosphate-binding drugs since the iron will be bound in the gut and not absorbed, rendering both treatments ineffective. The iron requirements in anaemic patients undergoing haemodialysis are often enormous and therefore IV iron is preferable mode of iron supplementation. IV iron e.g. iron saccharate 100 mg IV weekly is routine for patients with renal insufficiency unless ferritin above 800. This type of iron rarely causes a reaction unlike iron dextran.

Patients on CAPD may receive IV iron once monthly or in other intervals over 2 hours (iron sucrose, iron gluconate) according to patient's weight: if under 40 kg give 200 mg; 40–70 kg give 300 mg; over 70 kg give 500 mg.

If allergic reaction or anaphylactic shock occurs, stop infusion; give chlorpheniramine (Piriton) 10 mg IV over 1 min or hydrocortisone 100 mg IV or 0.5 ml of 1:1000 adrenaline IM (See Anaphylactic shock!).

Patients on haemodialysis can receive IV iron on dialysis at any time during the procedure. The ferritin level determines the frequency of iron administration:

Ferritin <100 µg/l: IV iron twice weekly;
Ferritin 100–300 µg/l: IV iron weekly;
Ferritin 300–600 µg/l: IV iron fortnightly.

Erythropoietin (rHuEPO):

Contraindication: malignant or poorly controlled hypertension. The rare complication of pure red cell aplasia is causing concerns at the moment: this is due to the production of neutralizing antibodies to erythropoietin and may depend on the precise formulation of erythropoietin and its route of administration. In order to avoid erythroblastopenia some centres use only IV erythropoietin, i.e. they do not use SC erythropoietin. Immunosuppressive treatment with corticosteroids, corticosteroids plus cyclophosphamide or ciclosporin accelerates recovery from erythropoietin-induced pure red cell aplasia.

Exclude conditions that result in unresponsiveness to erythropoietin such as iron deficiency (by far the commonest cause), hyperparathyroidism, chronic inflammation, deficiency of B12/folate, neoplasia (occult blood loss).

Starting dose of EPO 50 – 100 u/kg/week IV in three divided doses; SC dose is 30 – 50% less. In practice one usually starts with 1000u 3x/week SC, e.g. after dialysis and increase as necessary every month. Round the dose to the nearest 500 u. Increase the EPO dose every 6–8 weeks by 50% for Hct <30 or by 25% for Hct <33 until Hct 34 – 36%. If Hct >36% decrease the EPO dose by 20%.

Monitor Hb once monthly and iron studies once in 3 months.

Reduce the dose of EPO if Hb over 12 g/dl

Dosage guidelines for SC maintenance dose of EPO:

Weight <50 kg:	1000U + 1000U + 2000U per week
Weight 50–77 kg	2000U + 2000U + 2000U per week
Weight 75–100 kg	2000U + 2000U + 4000U per week
Weight >100 kg	2000U + 4000U + 4000U per week

A second generation erythropoetin agent, darbepoetin alfa has been granted a licence for treating anemia of chronic renal insufficiency. Clinical trials conducted on darbepoetin alfa have demonstrated success with once-weekly and once every other week dosing. Inject darbepoetin alfa by the same route of administration as previous rHuEpo (IV or SC). Patients receiving rHuEpo two or three times a week switch to darbepoetin alfa once a week, and those receiving rHuEpo once a week switch to darbepoetin alfa once every two weeks.

The average dose of darbepoetin alfa in patients with chronic kidney disease is 0.45 micrograms/kg once weekly or 0.75 micrograms/kg once every other week. The dose should be titrated to achieve and maintain a haemoglobin target concentration.

In some patients rHuEPO and iron replacement therapy are not sufficient to correct anemia. Folate deficiency may be a contributory factor in hyporesponsiveness to rHuEPO. Low red blood cell folate concentration in these patients indicates the need for folate supplementation (folic acid 5–15 mg od PO).

Adequate control of fluid balance in dialysis patients is easier if anemia is fully controlled!

Antibiotic prescriptions in CRI

Most antibiotics prescribed to patients in CRF are given in reduced doses (See Drug prescription in chronic renal failure). Trough (pre-dose) blood level should be checked for Vancomycin and aminoglycosides. Practical procedures for the administration of some antibiotics may be as follows:

Vancomycin 1 g in 100 ml normal saline given IV over 100 min every 48 hours, check trough blood level; should not be > 10 mg/L. Use for gram positive bacteria and in methicillin resistant staphylococcus aureus (MRSA);

Gentamicin: IM or by slow IV injection/infusion; loading dose 2 mg/kg IV followed by 60 mg/d (if b.w. <60 kg) or 80 mg/d (if b.w. >60 kg) od; trough level up to 2 mg/l. Use for gram negative microorganisms.

The dose of Ceftazidime is 1 g od, and for Cefuroxime 500–700 mg bd.

Nitrofurantoin is considered contra-indicated in renal failure.

Dietary modification

The minimal amount of dietary protein and calories required by normal adults or those with uncomplicated chronic renal insufficiency is 0.6 g of protein per day and 30–35 kcal/kg per day. Salt and protein restriction is difficult to achieve and severe protein restricted diets pose the risk of causing malnutrition. Protein restriction may reduce rate of RI progression by about 0.5 ml/min/year. Phosphate tends to be associated with protein so it is difficult to reduce phosphate levels in diet: phosphate absorption can be reduced by encouraging patients to take phosphate-binding drugs with all food.

Phosphate binders (eg calcium carbonate 300–1200 mg tds PO at start of meals). Other options include calcium acetate and sevelamer. Aluminium compounds are very effective phosphate binders but became unpopular because of aluminium toxicity in patients with renal failure. This is much less common when aluminium content of dialysis water is controlled (eg by reverse osmosis). There has been recent concern about the role of calcium-containing medications in promoting vascular calcification. Vitamin D3 analogues to suppress hyperparathyroidism (Alfacalcidol 0.25 μg three times a week as starting dose or Calcitriol 2 μg twice weekly PO at bedtime).

Hepatitis B vaccination

Check Hepatitis B and C serology and vaccinate if Hepatitis B negative. Uraemic patients respond poorly to vaccination and seroconversion rates are improved by early vaccination. We recommend vaccination in all patients likely to need dialysis in the future when their plasma creatinine is about 200 micromol/l. All staff members working in dialysis units should also be vaccinated.

The preparation we recommend for renal patients is HB Vax II 40 (1 dose = 1 ml). Note that there is also a HB-Vax II on the market but we recommend HB Vax II 40 so it is important to specify this precisely in the prescription. Injections are each 1 ml by IM injection, preferably into the deltoid muscle. Schedule is 1st dose of 1 ml IM at time 0, 2nd dose of 1 ml IM one month later, 3rd dose of 1 ml IM five months after the second dose. Approximately two months later, a serum sample is checked for anti-hepatitis B antibody. Patients who fail to respond should have a repeat course. Patients who make an inadequate response should have a booster dose or a complete repeat course. Routine boosters (1 ml IM) should be given at two year intervals.

Hyperlipidaemia

Hyperlipidaemia is common and it may be one of components in the multifactorial aetiology of cardiovascular disease that has a high incidence in patients with CRI. Advise patients to make an effort in weight reduction if she/he is overweight, suggest diet low in saturated fat.

Give statins if cholesterol and triglycerides are high e.g. atorvastatin 10–40 mg od PO. Check CPK (creatine phosphokinase) as rhabdomyolysis has been detected in a very small number of patients. Role of fibrates in renal failure is controversial: some think they reduce renal function and we do not recommend their use.

Hyperphosphataemia

Reduce phosphate in diet if possible.
Start phosphate binders when serum PO4 is above 1.8 mmol/l, sometimes at GFR 50–80 ml/min.

For patients with low serum calcium, high serum phosphate and high parathyroid hormone give phosphate binders: Calcichew 1.25 g tds (just before meals) or Calcichew forte or Titralac (1 Calcichew = 3 Titralac = 0.5 Calcichew Forte)

For patients with normal serum calcium, high phosphate and high PTH give Sevelamer 403 mg capsules, start 2 caps tds with meals and increase the dose according to plasma phosphate concentration to 3–4 caps tds. Alternatively use 1–2 caps of 800 mg with meals (tds).

Once Ca x P normal, and if PTH still raised, start initially with small dose of Alfacalcidol/calcitriol.

Hyperparathyroidism

Start Alfacalcidol when PTH is 3x upper limit of normal (actual numbers depend on assay used and normal range). Some specialists prefer pulse doses of calcitriol 2 µg twice weekly at bedtime: these may be better in patients with borderline tertiary hyperparathyroidism and are said to delay the need for parathyroidectomy.

Indications for parathyroidectomy include failure to suppress parathyroids without causing hypercalcaemia. Pre-operatively 2– 5 days loading with 4 µg Alfacalcidol PO and oral calcium (calcium-Sandoz 20 ml qds, or calcichew 1.25 g.

Following parathyroidectomy patient may become hypocalcaemic. Blood calcium concentration (ideally ionised calcium levels) should be measured immediately after the operation and frequently thereafter (up to four times per day for the first few postoperative days). Intravenous calcium is indicated if the patient develops rapid and progressive fall in serum calcium or develops symptoms related to hypocalcaemia or a plasma calcium concentration below 7.5 mg/dl (1.9 mmol/l). Initially, 10 ml of 10% calcium gluconate diluted in 50 ml of 5 percent dextrose should be infused over 10 to 20 minutes. Afterwards add 6–8 ampoules of 10 ml 10% calcium gluconate to 1 litre of 5% dextrose and infuse over 24 hours.

Maintain serum calcium concentration over 2 mmol/l with calcium gluconate, oral calcium supplements, Alfacalcidol 1–5 µg/day or calcitriol 2–4 µg/day.

Dialysis is another method capable of raising serum calcium levels. A high calcium bath (3.5 mEq/l) can be used in patients undergoing haemodialysis to ameliorate the severity of hypocalcaemia. Similarly, one to three 10 ml ampoules of 10% calcium gluconate can be added to each bag of peritoneal dialysate in patients treated with continuous ambulatory peritoneal dialysis.

The plasma phosphate and magnesium concentrations should also be monitored, since hypomagnesaemia can contribute to the development of refractory hypocalcaemia. Thus, raising the plasma magnesium concentration may contribute to correction of the hypocalcaemia.

Pregnancy

In pregnant women with chronic renal disease, dialysis should be considered earlier than in the non-pregnant patient. No evidence exists to support the superiority of one dialysis modality over another with respect to pregnancy outcome.

Haemodialysis sessions should be increased to 5–7 per week, with minimal heparinization and slow ultrafiltration to avoid dialysis hypotension and volume contraction.

If PD is used, decrease exchange volumes, and increase exchange frequencies. Anaemia should be corrected with iron, folic acid, and erythropoietin.

CLOSTRIDIUM DIFFICILE DIARRHOEA

Common in renal patients, who often have repeated exposures to broad spectrum antibiotics and frequent hospital admissions. Preventive methods include minimization of use of broad spectrum antibiotics especially cephalosporins, hand-washing and other measures to prevent cross-infection from affected individuals. Co-administration (with antibiotics) of Brewer's yeast has been advocated as a preventive treatment but has limited efficacy.

For proven or strongly suspected cases:
- Metronidazole 400 mg tds PO daily or
- Vancomycin 125 mg qds PO daily

each given for 7–14 days or until symptoms resolve and stool becomes negative for toxin of C. difficile.

COLIC (RENAL)

Nonsteroidal anti-inflammatory drugs (NSAIDs) have been used for pain control in patients with acute renal colic and are at least as effective as opiates, but in patients with pre-existing renal disease use these drugs with caution, for short time intervals and with as small as possible a dose as renal function may deteriorate.

When NSAID are used for renal colic, pain relief is achieved most rapidly by IV administration.

- Ketorolac trometamol initially 10 mg IM or IV over not less than 15 seconds, then 10–30 mg every 4–6 h PRN
- Indomethacin (100 mg) by rectal suppository
- Diclofenac 75 mg IM or 100 mg PR

Other drugs for renal colic:
- Paracetamol 0.5–1.0 gram up to 3 g per day
- Morphine sulphate 10 mg IV/IM/SC
- Pethidine 50 mg SC/IM or IV but do not use in Renal Insufficiency (use Morphine)
- Increase fluid intake

To reduce the risk of stone recurrence advise the patients to drink enough fluid to produce at least 2 litres of urine per day.

Patients whose stone have a low probability of spontaneous passage (on the basis of the size/localization) should be offered shock-wave lithotripsy, ureteroscopy with use of laser or percutaneous nephrolithotomy.

CONTRAST INDUCED NEPHROPATHY

Hydrate patient with isotonic saline 75–100 mL/h IV for 6 hours before and for 6 hours after procedure. Omit loop diuretics on day of procedure. Use low ionic contrast, minimise dose as much as possible without compromising efficiency of imaging procedure.

Acetylcysteine 600 mg bd PO may have some protective efficacy, administered for two days (24 hours before procedure and on the day of procedure).

CORTICOSTEROIDS

Many renal diseases are treated with high doses of corticosteroids (see also entries under individual categories especially "Glomerulonephritis"). Prednisolone is the form usually used for oral administration. 5 mg of prednisolone has equivalent anti-inflammatory potency to 6 mg of deflazacort, 20 mg of hydrocortisone, 4 mg of methyl prenisolone, 4 mg of triamcinolone or 750 micrograms of dexamethasone.

In patients receiving high doses of corticosteroids, we routinely advise gastric protection with a proton pump inhibitor eg omeprazole 10–40 mg daily PO or a H2 antagonist eg ranitidine 150 mg bd PO. We also routinely advise prophylaxis against steroid-induced osteoporosis. Bisphosphonates have been shown to be effective in renal transplant recipients and a convenient preparation is Fosamax Once-Weekly 70 mg per week (alendronate). Although the manufacturer recommends caution in patients with renal failure, we have found this preparation to be generally well-tolerated. Other bisphosphonate preparations may be equally effective.

CRAMPS (muscle cramps in CRF or dialysis patients)

Minimize interdialytic weight gain.
Prevent hypotension on dialysis including measures such as:
Infusion of saline
Infusion of 50% dextrose (25–50 ml)
Infusion of 10% mannitol 50–100 ml
Higher dialysate sodium concentration.
Quinine sulphate 300 mg at bed time PO.
Carnitine supplementation 20 mg/kg after each dialysis session or 1 g daily PO (1 g/10 mL single dose bottle)
Vit E 400 u od PO
Exercise, local massage of affected muscle.

DEEP VENOUS THROMBOSIS AND PULMONARY EMBOLISM (DVT AND PE) See: ANTICOAGULATION

DEPRESSION

The choice of the class or individual antidepressant drug depends on the patient's requirements. We will mention only a few frequently used and preferred drugs. From the class of tricyclic antidepressants: Amitriptyline hydrochloride 10 mg od PO or Lofepramine 70 mg od PO. From the class of selective serotonin re-uptake inhibitors: Fluoxetine 20 mg od PO.

DIABETES MELLITUS (DM)

Control of blood pressure (BP)

Once the presence of microalbuminuria is confirmed, initiate therapy with either ACEI or AIIRA, even if the patient is normotensive. In hypertensive diabetics aim to lower blood pressure to <130/80 mm Hg. For persons who have proteinuria of greater than 1 g/d and/or renal insufficiency regardless of aetiology, lower blood pressure to target of 125/75 mm Hg. Control of hypertension especially with ACEI or AIIRA reduces proteinuria and slows down progression of renal insufficiency. However, it is quite difficult to achieve these targets in everyday practice.

Begin therapy with a starting dose of drug, increasing the dosage as needed, to the high-dose range to achieve the blood pressure goal. Begin the therapy with one of ACEI's:

Enalapril 2.5 mg od, maintenance dose 10–20 mg od PO, max. 20 mg bd PO
Fosinopril 10 mg od, maintenance dose 10–40 mg od PO, max. 40 mg od PO
Lisinopril 2.5 mg od, maintenance dose 10–20 mg od PO, max. 40 mg od PO.
Perindopril 2 mg od, maintenance dose 4 mg od PO, max. 8 mg od PO.
Ramipril 1.25 mg od, maintenance dose 2.5–5 mg od PO, max. 10 mg od PO

Substitute ACEI with Angiotensin –II receptor antagonist if the patient has a persistent cough as a side effect of ACEI:

Candesartan 2 mg od PO, maintenance dose 8 mg od PO, max.16 mg od PO.
Irbesartan 150 mg od, max. 300 mg od PO
Losartan 25 mg od, usually 50 mg od PO, max. 100 mg od PO.
Valsartan 40 mg od PO, usually 80 mg od PO.

Dual therapy with ACEI and ARB is reasonable in patients in whom an optimal antiproteinuric effect (< 1 g protein/day) or blood pressure lowering effect has not been achieved.

Measure serum creatinine and electrolytes 1 week after initiating ACEI/AIIRA and after each increase in dose!

If BP still not at 130/80 mm Hg

Add thiazide diuretic: if serum creatinine <1.8 mg/dl (158 µmol/l) or loop diuretic if serum creatinine >1.8 mg/dl (158 µmol/l)

If BP still not at 130/80 mm Hg

Add long acting calcium channel blocker. A non-dihydropyridine CCB is recommended for patients with proteinuria >300 mg/d and pulse rate >84/min:

> Verapamil 80–120 mg bd or Verapamil SR 120–240 mg od
> Diltiazem SR 90–120 mg bd or Diltiazem XL 120 mg od

Dihydropyridine CCB is an alternative for patients with proteinuria <300 mg/d or pulse rate <84/min:

> Nifedipine 5 mg bd– tds, Nifedipine LA 20, 30, 60 mg od;
> Nifedipine Retard 10–20 mg bd
> Amlodipine 5–10 mg od

If BP still not at 130/80 mm Hg
For patients with pulse rate >84/min add low dose-beta blocker or alpha-beta blocker

> Atenolol 25–50 mg od
> Labetalol 100 mg od
> Carvedilol 3.125–6.25 mg od
> Bisoprolol 5 mg od
> Metoprolol 50–100 mg bd

Note that use of a beta-blocker with a nondihydropyridine CCB should be avoided. Anti-hypertensive and anti-proteinuric effects of beta-blockers are better than dihydropyridine CCB.

If BP still not at 130/80 mm Hg

Add other agents such as alpha-adrenoreceptor blocker Doxazosin 1 mg od PO, increased to 2 mg od PO after 1–2 weeks, max. 16 mg od; Doxazosin XL 4 mg od PO, increased to 8 mg od PO after 4 weeks if necessary), minoxidil, clonidine, hydralazine or methyldopa. Note that clonidine should not be used with beta-blockers.

Control of glycaemia in type II DM with renal insufficiency (target HbA1c <7.5%)

Oral hypoglycaemics with long half-lives such as chlorpropamide should be avoided because of the risk of hypoglycemia. Shorter acting drugs such as tolbutamide may be used but generally drugs which are not renally excreted such as gliclazide (Diamicron initially 80 mg od PO or Diamicron MR 30 mg od PO) are preferable in patients with renal insufficiency. Metformin (500 mg initially at breakfast for 1 week, then 500 mg with breakfast and evening meal for 1 week and finally 500 mg tds PO) increases the risk of lactic acidosis and should not be used in patients with creatinine level >200 µmol/l. In diabetics with creatinine below this level, metformin could be used. The kidney metabolizes insulin; therefore the dose of insulin requirement falls as renal insufficiency progresses.

Diabetic foot

Good local wound care; extensive debridement and relief of pressure on the ulcer are important components of therapy for foot ulcers. Advise the patients on the importance of appropriate foot wear; trainers are a cheap but effective substitute providing they fit well.

Cultures of the ulcer should be taken by swab. Culture of material obtained from deep in the ulcer is often helpful in choosing antibiotic therapy. A prolonged course (10 to 12 weeks) of intravenous antibiotics is still standard therapy, but some patients can be treated successfully by hospitalization for intravenous antibiotic therapy for 48 hours until the culture results are available, followed by appropriate oral antibiotic therapy at home. Antibiotics or combinations of antibacterial agents that may be used are as follows:

Flucloxacillin 500 mg qds IV and benzylpenicillin 600 mg qds IV

Metronidazole 500 mg tds IV or metronidazole 400 mg tds PO
Augmentin 375 mg tds PO or 1 g tds IV
Ciprofloxacin 250–500 mg bd PO or ciprofloxacin 200–400 mg bd IV
Cephalexin 250 mg qds PO or 500 mg tds PO
Clindamycin 300 mg tds PO for two weeks.
G-CSF therapy for one week: it offers eradication of pathogens from the infected ulcer, quicker resolution of cellulitis, shorter duration of intravenous antibiotic treatment, and shorter hospital stay.

Diabetic ketoacidosis

Identify and correct underlying causes (infection etc).
Infuse 1 litre of isotonic saline over 30 min.
Dissolve 50 u soluble insulin in 50 ml isotonic saline and give STAT 10 ml (10 u soluble insulin), followed by 6 ml/hour. Afterwards administer short-acting insulin as per Insulin sliding scale:

Blood glucose (mmol/L)	**Insulin infusion rate (ml/h)**
<5	no insulin, call physician
5.1–10.0	1
10.1–15.0	2
15.1–20.0	3
>20.1	6 and call physician

Then
Infuse1 litre of isotonic saline (no added potassium) over 1 hour

Then
1 litre of isotonic saline over 2 h (add potassium chloride – See below)

Then (subject to frequent reassessment of patient's hydration status) 1 litre of isotonic saline over 4 hours (add potassium chloride – See below)

Then (subject to frequent reassessment of patient's hydration status) 1 litre of isotonic saline over 6 hours (add potassium chloride – See below)

Add potassium to all saline infusions (after the first infusion 1litre/h): if serum potassium is 3.5–5 mmol/L, add 20 mmol KCl/l to saline; if serum potassium is < 3.5 mmol/l, add 40 mmol KCl/L saline. However, do not give potassium IV until urine output has been restored!

Check blood glucose hourly as long as the patient is on Insulin sliding scale. When blood glucose is less than 15 mmol/l (250 mg/dl), change infusion to ½ isotonic saline + 5% Dextrose 100 – 200 mL/h.

If acidaemia is severe (blood pH < 7,0 in young patient or <7.15 in older patients), give small amount sodium bicarbonate 1.26% 300 ml over 30 minutes or rarely 8.4% sodium bicarbonate 1 ml/kg over 1 hour.

Heparin 5,000 u bd SC until patient mobile.

If there is an infection give: Cefuroxime or amoxicillin 250–500 mg tds IV + flucloxacillin 250 mg qds IV + metronidazole 500 mg tds PR

Hyperosmolar diabetic coma: Blood osmolarity = 2Na+2K+serum glucose + serum urea; normal range 280–300, if higher than 340 rehydrate with ½ normal (0.45%) or normal (0.9%) sodium chloride over 48 hours till normal range is achieved.

Diabetic neuropathy

The most important measure for the prevention and treatment of diabetic neuropathy is optimal glucose control. By mechanisms that are less clear than in the case of nephropathy, ACEI may also be beneficial in diabetic retinopathy and neuropathy. Patients with painful diabetic neuropathy should be treated with a tricyclic antidepressant drug (Amitriptyline 10 mg tds PO to 25 mg tds PO); serotonin inhibitor (Fluoxetine 20 mg od PO) and sequentially add topical capsaicin cream 0.075% applied topically four times daily over painful areas.

If neuropathic pain continues add a third drug, most often carbamazepine 100–200 mg bd PO. Gabapentin (300 mg od PO) is licensed for the treatment of neuropathic pain and is an effective alternative to a tricyclic antidepressant. Nonsteroidal anti-inflammatory drugs are effective in patients with musculoskeletal or joint abnormalities secondary to long-standing neuropathy (ibuprofen 600 mg qds PO) can lead to substantial pain relief in patients with diabetic neuropathy.

Insulin requirement

Insulin requirements fall as renal insufficiency progresses, and then may rise again once dialysis is commenced.

DIURETICS

Diuretic therapy potentates the antihypertensive effects of most other antihypertensive drugs. For this reason they should be added as a second-step agent if blood pressure is inadequately controlled with any other drug chosen as a first-line agent.

Thiazides at low doses are used in the treatment of hypertension and heart failure. Weak thiazide diuretics are ineffective in patients with renal insufficiency (serum creatinine >200 µmol/l).

Bendrofluazide 2.5 and 5 mg, od PO in the morning or on alternate days
Hydrochlorothiazide 12.5–25 mg od PO.

In patients with refractory oedema metolazone 5 mg od PO is a potent thiazide diuretic, most effective in combination with loop diuretics (see below).

Loop diuretics should be used in renal insufficiency, if needed they may be combined with thiazide, and in refractory edema with Metolazone.

Frusemide is the loop diuretic most frequently used; oral dose is 40 mg od (preferably morning), maintenance dose 20 mg od PO, increase to 40 or 80 mg od PO in resistant oedema. The equivalent IV dose of frusemide is one half of the oral dose. The dose of frusemide in nephrotic syndrome is usually 80–120 mg od PO; the dose in CRF is usually 160–240 mg od PO and much higher daily doses may occasionally be used in patients with ARF (see below).

Parenteral dose (IM or IV) IV is usually ½ of oral dose. IV frusemide should be given by slow IV injection over 30 min to prevent ototoxicity.

After bolus dose, frusemide can be administered as IV infusion in isotonic saline starting at 10 mg/h and if diuresis is not sustained the dose can be increased to 20–30 or 40 mg/h.

Potassium sparing diuretics: Amiloride 5 mg bd PO or 10 mg od PO; Spironolactone100–200 mg daily) should only be used with extreme caution in renal insufficiency.

Metolazone (5–10 mg od) is the distal convoluted tubule diuretic most frequently combined with loop diuretics. Metolazone is effective even when renal failure is present.

Distal convoluted tubule diuretic (thiazide) should be administered some time before loop diuretic (1 hour) to ensure that NaCl transport in the distal nephron is blocked when flooded with solute.

DRUG PRESCRIPTION IN CHRONIC RENAL FAILURE

The dose of many drugs should be altered in patients with renal insufficiency (depending on the GFR), peritoneal and hemodialysis. The following table illustrates this for some frequently used drugs (cr.cl = creatinine clearance as estimate of excretory renal function, normal range 80–120 ml/min):

Drug	Renal Failure dose
ACE inhibitors and AIIRA	start with lowest dose; monitor serum creatinine and potassium.
Acetaminophen	no change
Acyclovir	reduce dose
Albuterol	reduce to 50% of normal dose
Allopurinol	reduce to 25% of normal dose; in severe RF only 100 mg/d or 100 mg on alternate days
Alendronic acid	manufacturer advises avoid if cr.cl. <35 ml/min
Amikacin	see aminoglycosides
Amiloride	monitor plasma K+, high risk of hyperkalaemia; avoid in severe RF
Aminoglycosides	reduce dose to 20 – 30%of normal dose/24 – 48 h, monitor serum conc.
Amiodarone	no change
Amitriptyline	no change
Amlodipine	no change
Amphotericin B	avoid, use only if no alternative

Ampicillin	reduce dose in severe RF
Atenolol	reduce (see beta-blockers)
Atorvastatin	caution if doses > 10 mg/d
Azithromycin	no change
Bendrofluazide	see thiazides
Benzylpenicillin	max 6 g/d. High doses may cause convulsions.
Beta-blockers	start with small dose, reduce dose in severe RF
Bezafibrate	reduce to 25% of normal dose, avoid in severe RF
Bisoprolol	reduce to 50% of normal dose
Bromocriptine	no change
Budesonide	no change
Bumetanide	no change, may need high doses
Carbamazepine	no change
Cefaclor	reduce 50% if cr.cl. <10 ml/min
Cefalexin	reduce, max 500 mg/d, dose after HD
Cefotaxime	reduce, loading dose 1 g/d then use ½ of normal dose
Ceftazidime	reduce to 1 g/48 h (1 g after HD) 0.5 g/d for CAPD
Ceftriaxone	reduce in severe RF
Cefuroxime	reduce in severe RF
Chloroquine	reduce to 50% of normal dose, avoid in severe RF
Chlorpheniramine	no change
Chlorpromazine	no change, start with small doses
Chlorpropamide	avoid
Cyclosporin	no change, monitor blood levels
Cimetidine	reduce to 600–800 mg/d, in severe RF 400 mg/d
Ciprofloxacin	reduce to ½ of normal dose
Clarithromycin	reduce to ½ of normal dose
Clindamycin	no change
Clonazepam	no change
Clonidine	no change
Clopidogrel	manufacturer advises caution

Codeine	reduce to 50%. Drug and metabolites may progressively accumulate
Colchicine	reduce to 50%
Co-trimoxazole	use 50% normal dose if cr.cl. 15–30 ml/min, avoid if cr.cl. <15 ml/min
Cyclophosphamide	reduce dose &/or adjust to keep total WBC >3.5x10^9/l, neutrophils >2.0x10^9/l
Desferrioxamine	no change
Dexamethasone	no change
Diamorphine	reduce dose
Diazepam	no change, but start with small dose
Diclofenac	see NSAID
Digitoxin	50–75% normal dose
Digoxin	10–25% normal dose/48 h
Diltiazem	no change but start with small dose
Dipyridamole	no change
Doxazosin	no change
Doxycycline	no change
Erythromycin	reduce to 50–75% in severe RF
Etidronate sodium	avoid (excreted by the kidney)
Felodipine	no change
Fluconazole	reduce maintenance dose by 50% if cr.cl. 20–50 ml/min and by 75% if cr.cl. <20 ml/min
Fluoxetine	reduce dose, avoid in severe RF
Fluvastatin	avoid in severe RF
Fosinopril	see ACE inhibitors
Frusemide	no change, may need high doses
Gabapentin	reduce dose
Ganciclovir	reduce dose
Gemfibrozil	no change
Gentamicin	reduce to 20–30%/24–48 h, monitor trough level
Glibenclamide	avoid, risk of hypoglycaemia
Gliclazide	reduce dose, less danger of hypoglycaemia as it is metabolized in the liver

Glipizide	increased risk of hypoglycaemia, avoid in severe RF
Haloperidol	no change, start with small doses
Heparin	no change, but increased risk of bleeding in severe RF (***LMW heparin)
Hydralazine	reduce dose if cr.cl. <30 ml/min
Hydrochlorothiazide	see Thiazides
Hydrocortisone	no change
Ibuprofen	see NSAID
Imipenem	reduce dose
Indapamide	see Thiazides
Indomethacin	see NSAID
Insulin	insulin requirements fall in CRF
Interferon alfa	avoid in severe RF
Ipratropium	no change
Isoniazid	reduce dose by 50% (max. 200 mg/d)
Isosorbide	no change
Isradipine	no change
Itraconazole	reduce to 50% (100 mg/d)
Kanamycin	reduce dose and frequency of maintenance doses, monitor trough serum concentrations and renal function
Ketoconazole	no change
Labetalol	no change
Lamivudine	reduce dose
Lansoprazole	no change
Levofloxacin	usual initial dose then 50% of normal dose
Lisinopril	see ACE inhibitors
Lithium carbonate	reduce the dose (25–50% and in renal replacement therapy 75%). Monitor plasma concentration. Avoid if possible.
Lorazepam	no change, but start with small dose
Losartan	see ACE inhibitors and AIIRA
Melphalan	reduce dose to 50%

Meropenem	mild RF 500 mg bd; moderate RF 250 mg bd; severe RF 250 mg od
Mesalazine	avoid in severe RF
Metformin	avoid (increased risk of lactic acidosis)
Methotrexate	relatively contraindicated when s.creatinine >2 mg/dL (>177 µmol/l). If unavoidable, use small dose at weekly or fortnightly intervals, monitor FBC carefully and watch for mucositis
Methyldopa	start with small dose
Methyl prednisolone	no change
Metoclopramide	avoid in severe RF
Metolazone	no change. See Thiazides (metolazone is effective in RF but risk of excessive diuresis)
Midazolam	start with 50% normal dose
Minoxidil	no change
Morphine	50% normal dose
Mycophenolate mofetil	caution and careful monitoring of WBC count
Nalidixic acid	ineffective in RF
Naloxone	no change
Naproxen	see NSAID
Nifedipine	no change
Nitrofurantoin	avoid
Nitroglycerine	no change
Nitroprusside	no change, avoid prolonged use.
Norfloxacin	½ normal dose if cr.cl. <30 ml/min, avoid in severe RF
NSAID	In mild RF, use lowest effective dose & monitor renal function. Avoid if possible in severe RF
Omeprazole	no change
Ondansetron	no change
Paroxetine	usual starting dose, small increments
Perindopril	see ACE inhibitors
Pethidine	do not use in RI (use morphine if needed)

Phenobarbitone	avoid large doses
Phenytoin	no change
Prazosin	start with 500 micrograms daily, increase with caution
Prednisolone	no change
Prednisone	no change
Pyrazinamide	use with caution
Quinine	reduce (see Malaria treatment and dose for renal failure)
Ramipril	see ACE inhibitors
Ribavirin	50% normal dose
Rifampicin	no change
Sertraline	manufacturer advises caution
Sildenafil	initial dose 25 mg if cr.cl. <30 ml/min
Simvastatin	no change, but in severe RF doses above 10 mg/d should be used with caution
Sotalol	reduce dose. See beta-blockers.
Spironolactone	monitor plasma K+, high risk of hyperkalaemia; avoid in severe RF
Streptokinase	no change
Streptomycin	reduce to one dose every 72–96 h in RF or ½ dose after each HD
Tamoxifen	no change
Tazocin	reduce dose if cr.cl. <30 ml/min. High sodium content
Temazepam	no change, start with small dose
Thiazides	avoid (ineffective in moderate or severe RF with exception of metolazone)
Trimethoprim	use ½ normal dose if cr.cl. <30 ml/min, avoid if cr.cl. <10 ml/min
Valacyclovir	reduce dose
Vancomycin	reduce dose and frequency - monitor plasma trough level
Verapamil	no change

ECLAMPSIA

Magnesium sulphate IV 4 g (4x2 ml of 2 mmol/ml, or 1 g/2 ml approximately 16 mmol Mg^{2+}) over 5–10 minutes followed by IV infusion at a rate of 1 g (approximately 4 mmol Mg^{2+}) every hour for at least 24 hours after the last seizure. Urgent delivery!

EPILEPSY

Generally, management is as for non-renal patients. Non-convulsive status epilepticus is more common in patients with renal failure and should be considered in any patient with unexplained impairment of consciousness.

Drug therapy:
Carbamazepine (Tegretol) start with 100 mg/12 h PO
Sodium valproate (Epilim): start with 200 mg/12 hours, PO max 30 mg/kg/24 hours.
Phenytoin 150–300 mg daily as a single dose or in two divided doses
Phenobarbitone 60–180 mg at night, 200 mg IM and in status epilepticus 10 mg/kg at a rate of not more than 100 mg/min, max. 1 g.

Diazepam is often considered the drug of first choice in status epilepticus. IV diazepam can cause thrombophlebitis: this is minimized by using the emulsion formulation (Diazemuls). Dose is 10-20 mg IV at a rate of 2.5 mg every 30 seconds until a response is achieved. The dose can be repeated if necessary after 30–60 minutes. Facilities for mechanical ventilation should be at hand in case of respiratory depression. Diazepam can also be administered as a rectal solution (500 micrograms/kg) if IV access is not available. The reversal agent flumazenil should be available.

ERECTILE DYSFUNCTION

Sildenafil (Viagra) should be used at reduced dose in renal impairment, initial dose 25 mg if creatinine clearance <30 ml/min. Contra-indications: treatment with nitrates, hypotension (systolic BP < 90 mmHg).
Apomorphine 100 mg PO one hour before intercourse
Reversal of anaemia with erythropoietin improves sexual function in some patients.

It is important to know about the aetiology of erectile dysfunction as well as the mechanisms by which drugs may improve erection in order to decide which drug is appropriate for a particular patient. Intracorporal pharmacotherapy is an alternative if no response to oral agent is achieved. Various mechanical devices are also available.

ETHYLENE GLYCOL INTOXICATION

(Identical treatment for Methanol poisoning)

Prompt treatment is required to prevent death or permanent tissue injury. Many aspects of therapy are similar with methanol and ethylene glycol.

Gastric lavages should be performed if the patient is seen in the first few hours after drug ingestion to minimize further drug absorption. Charcoal administration may further reduce absorption.

Sodium bicarbonate should be given to correct the metabolic acidosis. Massive doses of sodium bicarbonate may be required if the acidosis is severe and/or there is continuing acid production.

Fomepizole rapidly and competitively inhibits alcohol dehydrogenase more potently than ethanol, but without the toxicity and with fewer adverse side effects. Therefore it is now first-line therapy and the antidote of choice in cases of methanol and ethylene glycol intoxication. Treatment with fomepizole should be initiated as quickly as possible when there is a suspicion of methanol or ethylene glycol poisoning. A loading dose of 15 mg/kg should be given in 100 ml of 5% dextrose over 30 minutes, followed by boluses of 10–12 mg/kg every 12 hours for 48 hours, then 15 mg/kg every 12 hours thereafter until methanol or ethylene glycol concentrations fall below 20 mg/dl.

Intravenous or oral ethanol is an essential component of early therapy in these disorders unless fomepizole is administered. Alcohol dehydrogenase, the enzyme responsible for the formation of toxic metabolites, has more than a 10-fold greater affinity for ethanol than for other alcohols. The efficacy of ethanol is most prominent when the plasma ethanol concentration is about 100 to 200 mg/dL (22 to 33 mmol/l). This level can generally be achieved by the following regimen: a loading dose of 0.6 g/kg plus an hourly maintenance dose of 66 mg/kg in nondrinkers, 154 mg/kg in drinkers, and 240 mg/kg once hemodialysis is started. If oral ethanol is given, the dose may have to be doubled if charcoal has been administered. Regardless of the mode of administration, the plasma ethanol concentration should be monitored, since adjustments in dosage will be required in some patients. Ethanol and, if necessary, hemodialysis are continued until a low plasma drug level is achieved; for example, less than 10 to 20 mg/dl (3 to 6 mmol/l) with methanol intoxication.

Ethanol can be given in a variety of different solutions. Intravenous ethanol comes in 5 or 10 percent solutions (5 or 10 g per 100 ml) diluted in dextrose and water. Oral or nasogastric ethanol is usually given as a 20 percent solution, which can be created by adding 21 ml of 95 percent ethanol to 79 ml of water or another tolerable diluent. Different whiskies vary in concentration from 90 proof (45 percent) to 190 proof (95 percent).

Haemodialysis is a part of treatment because in addition to stopping the metabolism of ethylene glycol with Fomepizole or ethyl alcohol, we have to remove ethylene glycol. Therefore, it should be performed in severe intoxications to remove both the parent compound and metabolites. The haemodialysis prescription should include a large surface area dialyzer (>1.5 m^2), a blood flow rate in excess of 300 ml/min, and a a high concentration of bicarbonate in the bath. Drug removal is much slower with peritoneal dialysis (due to the lower flow rates); as a result, this modality should be used only if haemodialysis is not available.

General indications for haemodialysis have included a high plasma level (more than 50 mg/dl or 15 mmol/l for methanol or more than 20 mg/dl for ethylene glycol), the presence of metabolic acidosis, and symptoms (such as visual or mental status changes with methanol). Haemodialysis is continued until the plasma levels fall below the toxic range.

Fomepizole is dialyzable and the frequency of its dosing should be increased in patients on haemodialysis. An additional dose should be given at the beginning of haemodialysis if 6 hours have elapsed since the prior dose.

Several other modalities may be beneficial: folic acid (50 to 70 mg IV every four hours for the first day); pyridoxine (50 mg IM, four times daily) and thiamine (100 mg IM, four times daily).

In addition, a forced diuresis with fluids and mannitol may preserve renal function during ethylene glycol intoxication by minimizing tubular blockade by oxalate crystals.

FLUID (for IV administration)

Fluid replacement should be guided by an approximate calculation of amounts of fluid and salt lost, preceded by accurate clinical assessment ± invasive measurements (CVP or PCWP) and monitored by frequent repeat assessments. A reasonable regimen in mildly hypovolaemic patients is 3 litres of IV fluid/d; usually 2 litres of isotonic saline and 1 litre of 5% Dextrose. If patient has low potassium add 20 mEq potassium/litre of IV fluid. Start at 60 ml/h and increase if needed to 80 or 100 ml/h. Check urine output.

Sodium chloride: isotonic (0.9%, normal) saline
Glucose intravenous infusion 5% (5% Dextrose)
Human albumin solution 4.5% (50, 100, 250, 400 ml)
Human albumin solution 5% (50, 100, 250, 400 and 500 ml bottles)
Human albumin solution 20% (10, 50 and 100 ml vials/bottles)
Gelatin (Gelofusine, Haemaccel) solution 500 ml IV to keep CVP 8–10 mm (if CVP line is inserted!).

GLOMERULAR FILTRATION RATE (GFR)

Can be accurately measured by injection of a tracer amount of radioisotope (usually ^{51}chromium-labelled EDTA) and measurement of residual radioactivity in blood at timed intervals (usually 1, 2, 3 and 4 hours) after injection. Rate of decline is proportional to GFR since EDTA is freely filtered by the glomerulus and not reabsorbed. Urine collection/testing is not required for this test.

Estimations of GFR can be made by creatinine clearance (CrCl). This can be measured by collecting urine for a timed period (usually 24 hours), measurement of urine creatinine concentration and simultaneous plasma creatinine concentration and calculation according to the formula UV/P (urine concentration X urine flow rate in ml/min, divided by plasma concentration). However, we rarely advocate urine collections for assessment of creatinine clearance since they are notoriously unreliable. We prefer to calculate creatinine clearance from the plasma creatinine, correcting for gender, age and body weight, eg using the Cockroft-Gault formula:

For males:
CrCl (in ml/min) = 1.23 X (140-age) X weight in kg, divided by plasma creatinine in micromol/l

For females:
CrCl (in ml/min) = 1.04 X (140-age) X weight in kg, divided by plasma creatinine in micromol/l

GLOMERULONEPHRITIS (GN)

Acute poststreptococcal glomerulonephritis

Therapy for patients with APSGN is symptomatic and depends on the clinical severity of the illness. The major aims are to control the oedema and blood pressure.

During the acute phase of the disease, salt and water should be restricted. If significant oedema or hypertension develops, diuretics should be administered. Loop diuretics increase urinary output and consequently improve cardiovascular congestion and hypertension.

For hypertension not controlled by diuretics, calcium channel blockers or angiotensin-converting enzyme inhibitors are generally useful. For malignant hypertension, intravenous nitroprusside or other parenteral agents are used.

The indications for dialysis include life-threatening hyperkalaemia and clinical manifestations of uraemia. In patients with rapidly progressive renal failure, a renal biopsy is indicated. If the biopsy shows crescentic glomerulonephritis with more than 30% of the glomeruli involved, a short course of intravenous pulse steroid therapy is recommended (500 mg–1 g/1.73 m^2 of methylprednisone od IV for 3–5 d).

Antiglomerular basement membrane (anti-GBM) disease, Goodpasture's disease

This is due to a pathogenic IgG autoantibody, and treatment has been rationally designed to deal with this. Corticosteroids to reduce inflammation provoked by deposited antibody, plasma exchange to remove pre-formed antibody from the circulation, cyclophosphamide to prevent further antibody synthesis. The main determinant of outcome is the extent of tissue damage at the time of initiation of therapy.

Methylprednisolone 0.5 g/day IV for three consecutive days, followed by prednisolone 1 mg/kg/day (maximum 60 mg/day) orally, decreasing by 10 mg/week until the dose of 20 mg is reached, then decrease by 2.5 mg/fortnight and withdraw after 6 months.

Plasma exchange, 4 l/day for at least 14 days or until assays for anti-GBM antibodies are persistently negative. Substitute fluid 4.5% human albumin. If bleeding tendency and/or recent tissue biopsy, at the end of exchange give 200–300 ml Fresh Frozen Plasma (FFP).

Cyclophosphamide 3 mg/kg/day PO (rounded down to nearest 50 mg). Reduce dose to 2 mg/kg/day in elderly (over 55 years) or in renal insufficiency. Stop cyclophosphamide when total WBC<3.5×10^9/l or neutrophil count < 2.0×10^9/l. Duration of therapy with Cyclophosphamide 2 months.

Renal recovery is unusual if advanced renal impairment is present at the time of diagnosis (patient dialysis-dependent or serum creatinine >500 µmol/L (>5.7 mg/dL) and some units would not treat such patients with aggressive immunosuppression. However, if pulmonary haemorrhage is associated, full treatment including plasma exchange is indicated irrespective of the likelihood of renal recovery.

Focal segmental glomerulosclerosis (FSGS)

The initial treatment for primary FSGS in adults is high dose of Prednisolone 1 mg/kg/day (up to 80 mg/day) for 8–12 weeks, followed by 0.5 mg/kg/day for 6–8 weeks, and then tapering to a stop over 8 weeks. Response may not be obtained in the first 2–4 months of therapy, some advocate even longer courses. If no response after 4–6 months consider alternative therapy.

In patients who relapse after a prolonged period off steroids (>6 months) a second course of steroid therapy could be sufficient.

In patients who are frequent relapsers, or steroid dependent or who do not tolerate steroids, the use of cytotoxic agents or cyclosporine has been beneficial. A course of cytotoxic agent (cyclophosphamide 2 mg/kg/day for 8–12 weeks or chlorambucil 0.1 to 0.2 mg/kg/day for 2 to 3 months) in combination with a low dose of steroids (prednisolone up to 30 mg/day) can be associated with a reduction of relapses and more prolonged remissions.

Steroid responsive patients who have frequent relapses may have a good response to Cyclosporin 3 – 5 mg/kg/day for 4–12 months. Monitor blood level (should be in the range 75–150 ng/ml).

Steroid resistant FSGS is difficult to treat; the use of cyclosporin results in more favourable responses than cytotoxic agents. Mycophenolate mofetil (start with 0.25 g bd PO and increase to 1 g bd) has been tried in small numbers of such patients. Continue therapy for at least 3–12 months.

ACEI or angiotensin II receptor blockers are used for control of proteinuria. Statins are used for control of hyperlipidaemia.

The use of plasmapheresis or immunoadsorption has been successful in the treatment of recurrent FSGS in renal transplant patients.

IgA nephropathy (Berger's disease)

In patients with low risk, i.e. proteinuria <1 g/day, treat only with ACEI or AIIRA even if they are normotensive in an attempt to reduce proteinuria. Maximally tolerated dose should be used, focusing on lowering protein excretion. Combination of an ACE inhibitor and an AIIRA may result in better for anti-proteinuric effect than either given alone.

In high-risk patients with proteinuria >1 g/day and elevated serum creatinine (1.5–3 mg/dl/or >133 μmol/l), in addition to ACEI for reduction of proteinuria as in other forms of nephropathy, there is no widely accepted form of therapy but various approaches have been suggested, based on combination of steroids and immunosuppressive agents:

(i) steroids: methylprednisolone 1 g "pulse dose" in 100 ml 5% dextrose or isotonic saline over at least 60 minutes for three consecutive days, followed by prednisolone 1 mg/kg/day for 2 months, than taper prednisolone to 0.6 mg/kg/d for 2 months followed by 0.3 mg/kg/d for an additional 2 months and finally reduce to maintenance dose of 10 mg/kg/day. Prolonged treatment (3 to 6 months) is required to obtain benefit.

(ii) immunosuppression:
- azathioprine 2 mg/kg/day od PO plus low dose prednisolone or

- cyclophosphamide 2 mg/kg/day orally or
- mycophenolate mofetil 0.25 g bd PO increasing to 1g bd PO
- and finally, for crescentic IgA nephropathy steroids as above plus pulse cyclophosphamide IV at 0.5–0.75 g/m^2 body surface area monthly for 6 months.

(iii) Fish oils ("Maxepa") 5 g two times a day PO with food may show beneficial effects (reduced progression to renal insufficiency) despite a lack of effect on proteinuria.

Membranous nephropathy

Exclude secondary causes.

Low-risk patients (proteinuria <4 g/day, normal renal function): conservative treatment: diet, normalize blood pressure with ACEI.

Medium-risk patients (proteinuria 4–8 g/day, normal renal function): ACEI, statin, consider prophylactic anticoagulation if plasma albumin less than 20 g/L.

High-risk patients (proteinuria > 8 g/day, abnormal renal function): consider immunosuppressive therapy (corticosteroids + cytotoxic agent or corticosteroids + cyclosporin).

Many centres use Ponticelli regimen or its modifications in the treatment of membranous nephropathy:

Month 1, 3 and 5: Methylprednisolone 1 g/day pulse dose IV for three consecutive days followed by oral prednisolone 0.5 mg/kg/day for 27 days.

Month 2, 4 and 6: Chlorambucil 0.1–0.2 mg/kg/day for 30 days (lower dose in patients over 50 years or if GFR less than 60; stop if total WBC<3.5×10^9/l or neutrophil count < 2.0×10^9/l).

Alternative protocol is with the use of oral cyclophosphamide 1.5 mg/kg/d PO instead of chlorambucil; this treatment may have fewer side-effects.

The other therapeutic options are: cyclosporin 3–5 mg/kg/day aiming initially for trough level 75–150 ng/ml combined with prednisolone 0.5 mg/kg/day (duration of therapy 6–12 months) or mycophenolate mofetil (MMF). Initiate MMF at 0.5 g bd and increase as tolerated to 1 g bd. Reduce the dose by 33% (1/3) in patients with reduced GFR or gastrointestinal side-effects. Discontinue MMF if total WBC decreased to <3.5x10^9/L or if liver enzymes increased to >2 times the upper limit of normal. In patients who respond dramatically within three months, consider discontinuation of treatment after six months. In those who relapse or in those whose maximal response takes three to six months to achieve, extend treatment period to at least one year.

Additional (adjunctive) therapy:

Diuretics to control edema.

ACEI for control of blood pressure, useful additional effect on reducing proteinuria

Statin for control of hyperlipidaemia! Statin may also reduce proteinuria.

Co-trimoxazole for prevention of Pneumocystis carinii infection

Bisphophonates to prevent bone loss on long-term steroid use

Anticoagulants to prevent renal vein thrombosis or DVT especially in patients who have suffered a venous thrombosis or a PE or have had prolonged period of massive proteinuria. Since patients with nephrotic syndrome due to membranous nephropathy are at high risk of intravascular thrombosis including renal vein thrombosis, evidence favours prophylactic anticoagulation with warfarin if plasma albumin is less than 20 g/l.

Rare cases of membranous nephropathy associated with hepatitis-B or C virus infections may resolve if anti-viral therapy is successful. Corticosteroids and immunosuppressive drugs are of limited value in these patients as they may enhance viral replication.

Maintain adequate nutrition!

Membranoproliferative glomerulonephritis (MPGN; synonymous with Mesangiocapillary GN, MCGN)

In children, some centres advocate high dose alternate day corticosteroids (eg prednisolone 2 mg/kg/ on alternate days PO until improvement noted, evidenced by reduction of proteinuria, a fall in serum creatinine concentration, then gradually reduced to maintenance dose of 20 mg PO on alternative days. Some centres would also try this treatment in adults but there is no evidence favouring this approach.

A combination of Dipyridamole 100 mg tds PO and Aspirin 300 mg od PO has been used in adults, but there is no evidence to support long-term efficacy of this treatment.

If cryoglobulinaemia is present, associated hepatitis C infection or lymphoproliferative disease should be sought and treated if positively identified. Cryoglobulinaemia can be treated with plasma exchange (usually daily 4 litre exchanges for 5 consecutive days will remove pre-formed cryoglobulin). In idiopathic cases (ie no evidence of hepatitis C or underlying lymphoproliferative disorder), initial maintenance treatment with steroids and cyclophosphamide is usually effective. Long-term maintenance treatment is more controversial: low dose chlorambucil, monthly plasma exchange, mycophenolate mofetil all may be useful in individual cases.

Additional therapy: ACEI to reduce proteinuria and to treat hypertension.

Mesangial non-IgA proliferative glomerulonephritis

(Without IgA deposits; IgM nephropathy; C1q nephropathy; associated with Lupus)

In patients with isolated hematuria or hematuria combined with proteinuria < 1g/d, no treatment other than management of hypertension is needed. In patients with nephrotic syndrome, even though there are no controlled trials, some nephrologists use an initial course of corticosteroids 1 mg/kg/d (prednisolone max. 60 mg/d) for 2–3 months followed by a lower dose for 2–3 additional months. Relapsing steroid-responsive patients may benefit from the addition of cyclophosphamide, chlorambucil or cyclosporin.

Minimal change disease

Prednisolone 1 mg/kg/day, max. 60 mg/day for 8–12 weeks or until remission. Remission is usually between days 7–14. Adults respond more slowly than children, some patients need up to 16 weeks of therapy to achieve complete remission. When proteinuria disappears, or 1 week after remission has been induced, continue prednisolone 0.5 mg/kg/d for another 6–8 weeks, then slowly taper over next 8 weeks aiming to stop the treatment.

If no response give pulses of methylprednisolone 1 g for 3 days, then prednisolone for 12 weeks.

If possible, give steroids on alternate days.

Second course of steroids could be given to patients with relapse.

If the patient is steroid resistant, steroid-dependent, has frequent relapses or if he/she cannot tolerate side effects of steroids, an alternative is Cyclophosphamide 1.5–2 mg/kg/day 8–12 weeks. Give concomitantly prednisolone 7.5–15 mg od PO. Check WBC count every 2 weeks; if total WBC<3.5×10^9/l or neutrophil count < 2.0×10^9/l stop cyclophosphamide until WBC/neutrophil recovery then re-start at ½ of original dose. The alternative to oral cyclophosphamide is IV pulse cyclophosphamide 500 mg/m^2 monthly for 6 months.

Other cytotoxic agents that may be used in the treatment of MCD are mycophenolate mofetil (0.25 g bd and increase the dose to 1 g bd) or chlorambucil (see Membranous nephropathy).

Cyclosporin and Tacrolimus are generally reserved for patients with MCD initially unresponsive to steroids or alkylating agents. It is usually necessary to give prolonged courses up to 1 year or longer as relapses are frequent after discontinuation of cyclosporine. Low doses of cyclosporine should be used (3–5 mg/kg/d). Blood level (trough) 80–150 ng/ml). Give concomitantly prednisolone 7.5–15 mg od PO.

HAEMODIALYSIS

Antibiotic prescribing in HD patients

Antibiotic	non-uremic dosage	Usual dosage in dialysis patient
Amoxicillin	500 mg TDS	500 mg BD
Cefotaxime	1–2 g QDS	1–2 g OD
Ceftazidime	0.5–2 g QDS/TDS	1 g every other day
Ceftriaxone	1–2 g OD	1 g OD
Cephradine	0.5 g QDS	250 mg BD.
Ciprofloxacin	500 mg BD	250 mg BD
Clarithromycin	250–500 mg BD	250 mg OD
Erythromycin	500 mg QDS	500 mg QDS
Imipenem	0.5–1 g QDS/TDS	125–250 mg OD
Metronidazole	500 mg TDS	250 mg TDS

HD Prescription (HD order)

Dialyser: various sizes available, start with lower size.
Dialyser surface area 0.7–1.4 m².
Start: 2 hrs dialysis time for first HD session, three hours second HD session and thereafter 4 hrs/session.
Blood flow at start 150 ml/min for 50 kg patients, 200 ml/min for 50–70 kg patient
Dialysate temperature 35–37 °C
Dialysate composition: to be determined according to blood biochemistry. On average, the composition is as follows:
Bicarbonate 25–40 mEq/l, standard 35 mEq/L, for acute renal failure 25 mEq/L
Mg 0.75–1.5 mEq/L, mean 0.5–1 mEq/L
Calcium 1–4, usually 2.5 mEq/L
Potassium 2–4.5 mEq/L, if serum potassium >5.5 use 2 mEq/l, for acute usually 3.5 mEq/L
If pre–HD serum K <4, use 4 mEq/L
Sodium 135–145 mEq/L, standard usage 140 mEq/L
Glucose 200 mg/dL (to prevent hypoglycemia)
Dialysate flow rate 500 ml/hr.
Fluid removal orders: depends upon blood pressure, target weight and inter-dialytic fluid gains. On average, can readily remove 2–2.5 L over 4 hours at a constant rate.
Anticoagulation order: heparin bolus 1000 – 2000 u, followed by heparin infusion into arterial blood line at a rate 1000–2000 u/h. For reversal of prolonged access bleeding protamine sulphate can be given IV 1 mg/100 units of heparin when given within 15 min of heparin; if longer time, less protamine sulphate is required as heparin is rapidly excreted.

Heparin free dialysis is the method used for patients who are actively bleeding or who are at high risk of bleeding (recent surgery). This technique is based on frequent saline rinses and high flow rate.

Low molecular weight heparin can also be used for anticoagulation during haemodialysis. Enoxaparin (Clexane) 0.7 mg/kg/session can be injected into arterial line pre-dialyser, 3–4 min before haemodialysis. For reversal of prolonged access bleeding protamine sulphate can be given in a dose 0.5–1 mg/mg of Enoxaparin IV.

HD catheter lock

Heparin 5,000 U into each limb of a-v line

HD catheter-related infections

The options for treatment (depending on the severity of infection, and signs of sepsis) are:
- leave catheter in and try antibiotic management;
- change catheter over guide wire;
- change catheter over guide-wire with a new tunnel and exit site;
- remove catheter and delay replacement until the infection has been treated.

Initiate treatment with empirical broad-spectrum antibiotics (vancomycin and gentamicin) immediately after taking blood for blood cultures through the catheter and from a peripheral vein. Infuse the loading dose of vancomycin 1 g during last hour of haemodialysis and give gentamicin 1.5 mg/kg immediately after completion of dialysis session. The maintenance doses to be given on dialysis sessions: vancomycin 500 mg and gentamicin 1 mg/kg, the dose should be altered according to trough drug levels. If the initial blood cultures result in no growth for five days, discontinue the antibiotics. All patients with positive blood cultures should be treated with IV antibiotics for three weeks. Once a pathogen is identified and antibiotic sensitivities available modify the antibiotic regimen accordingly.

Remove catheter if infection serious with signs of septicaemia, persistent fever, hemodynamic instability or tunnel infection.

However, removal of a tunneled dialysis catheter is not mandatory in all patients with documented sepsis. The instillation of antibiotic locks (highly concentrated antibiotic solution) into the catheter lumen after dialysis session in conjunction with systemic antibiotics appears to be effective and safe in a substantial number of patients. The dialysis lines are then 'locked' upon completion of each dialysis session with a solution containing:

1 mL vancomycin (5 mg vancomycin/mL of saline) + gentamicin 0.5 mL (gentamicin 4 mg/mL saline) + sodium citrate 1.5 mL of 3.8% solution (gentamicin is not compatible with heparin). The fluid used

to "lock" the catheter should always be withdrawn prior to next use, but it may be prudent to check blood levels of gentamicin at weekly intervals, taking blood through a peripheral site not through the catheter itself.

HD catheter thrombosis

The following procedures could be used for malfunctioning thrombosed catheter:

Saline flush: fill a 10 mL syringe (Luer lock) with saline, attach firmly to the catheter, and flush into the catheter with as much force as can be generated with the hand. Once done, an attempt to aspirate blood should be made. If no blood can be aspirated, the saline flush can be repeated several times. If blood can be aspirated, the procedure should be repeated multiple times using blood until flow seems to be free and easy.

Intraluminal lytic enzymes

a) Instillation of **Urokinase** 5000 IU/mL to the volume of the catheter. Aspirate after 30 min; repeat if unsuccessful. Similar solution can be instilled overnight if required.

b) **tPA** 10 mg vial, reconstitute with 0.9 percent saline to give a total volume of 10 mL or a concentration of 1 mg/mL. To treat a thrombosed catheter, 1 mg (1 mL) of thawed tPA is instilled into each lumen of the catheter and backed up with a quantity of saline so that the total volume equals the fill volume of the catheter. After being allowed to dwell for two hours, an attempt is made to aspirate the catheter. If the attempt is successful, 5 mL of blood is removed and discarded. The catheter is then flushed with 10 mL of saline. If the catheter is patent, the dialysis treatment is initiated. If the catheter remains occluded, a second dose of tPA is instilled in the same manner as previously. If, after two additional hours, this lytic therapy continues to be unsuccessful, the patient is sent for secondary treatment of his or her catheter thrombosis.

c) Reteplase may also be efficient in restoring flow to malfunctioning haemodialysis catheter: reteplase 0.4 u instill into each port; dwell time 30 sec. If aspiration is not possible, leave reteplase in the catheter for additional 30 sec. If flow was established (>200 mL/min) use catheter for haemodialysis.

Mechanical therapy: an endoluminal brush can be used to open dysfunctional hemodialysis catheters.

Catheter exchange over a guide-wire: Catheter exchange over a guidewire can be effectively used to eliminate intrinsic catheter thrombosis and is the secondary treatment of choice for intrinsic catheter thrombosis

Urokinase infusion: 200 micrograms/kg/hr in each port. Infuse for 6 h. Administration of this dose of urokinase does not result in systemic effects nor require hospital admission.

Hypertension in HD patients

Correct over-hydration (fluid overload) by an increase of dialysis time to achieve and maintain target "dry" weight. If blood pressure control still not adequate, step up to drug treatment:
- calcium channel blockers, especially long acting dihydropyridine: Amlodipine 5 mg od PO, Diltiazem XL 120, 180, 240 mg ; Diltiazem SR 60 mg 90, 120 mg od PO. Do not use short-acting formulation of nifedipine, as it may precipitate cerebral and myocardial infarction or retinal ischemia.
- ACEI: Enalapril 2.5, 5–20 mg od PO, Lisinopril 2.5, 5–20 mg od PO, Ramipril 1.25, 2.5–10 mg od PO, perindopril 2–4 mg od PO.
- angiotensin II receptor antagonists: Losartan 25–50 mg od PO, Candesartan 2–32 mg od PO.
- sympatholytic drugs: methyldopa 125–250 mg bd/tds; clonidine 50–100 micrograms tds PO (must be withdrawn gradually to avoid hypertensive crisis);
- take extreme caution with the use of vasodilator antihypertensive drugs: Hydralazine 25–50 mg bd PO; Minoxidil initially 2.5 mg od PO, increase (if needed) every third day by 2.5 mg, max. in non-dialysis patient 50 mg daily. This drug promotes salt and water retention.
- beta blockers (Atenolol 25 mg od PO, increase to max 100 mg od PO); alpha/beta blockers Carvedilol 5 mg od PO, Labetalol 100 mg bd PO, increase if needed to 200 mg bd PO;

- alpha blocker Doxazosin 1 mg od PO (at bedtime), increase if needed to 2 mg od PO or newer formulation doxazosin XL 4 mg/day and maximum dose 8 mg/day.

Hypertension at the end of HD may be due to sympathetic release and vasoconstriction. The drug of choice in this condition is alpha-blocker (Doxazosin 2 mg od PO).

Hypertensive emergency:
Nitroprusside continuous IV infusion 0.3–0.8 µg/kg/min not for longer than 48 hours. Labetalol IV (in patients without asthma or heart block) 50 mg IV over 1 min, repeat every 5 min, max 200 mg.

Hypophosphataemia

Phosphate Sandoz 1–2 tbl tds PO

Hypotension

The following procedures could be considered to treat or prevent episodes of hypotension during hemodialysis:
- The patient should be placed in the Trendelenburg position.
- Ultrafiltration should either be stopped or the rate decreased.
- The blood flow rate should be reduced.
- Intravenous bolus of saline is first-line therapy for hypotension.
- An increase of intravascular fluid volume may be achieved with IV mannitol.
- Increase dialysate sodium concentration and sodium modeling: the use of a constant higher dialysate sodium concentration (≥140 mEq/L) or a linear sodium ramping (155 to 140 mEq/L); or stepwise sodium ramping (155 mEq/L for three hours and 140 mEq/L for one hour).
- Cool dialysate to 35°C
- Isolated Ultrafiltration followed by isovolaemic dialysis
- Steady, constant ultrafiltration at a rate less than 0.3 ml/kg/min
- Sequential ultrafiltration and isovolaemic dialysis: initial ultrafiltration alone (without dialysis) followed by

- isovolaemic dialysis in which little or no further fluid removal occurs due to reduced transmembrane pressures.
- Increasing the dialysate calcium concentration.
- Avoid ingestion of a meal immediately before or during dialysis.
- Consider longer haemodialysis sessions
- Linear Ultrafiltration
- Oral Midodrine, an alpha-1 adrenergic agonist, 2–5 mg 30 min before hemodialysis

Recommendation for prevention of intradialytic hypotension

- Accurate setting of the "dry weight".
- Correction of anaemia with erythropoetin.
- Avoidance of food — food ingestion during dialysis leads to a significant decline in systemic vascular resistance that can contribute to a fall in blood pressure.
- Verapamil 40 mg od PO pre-dialysis
- Limit interdialytic weight gain and if weight gain was due to fluid intake, consider ACEI as useful antidipsogenic agents and restrict sodium intake
- Avoid short acting hypotensive agents evening before HD, morning before HD or shortly before HD.
- Consider whether the patient is below dry weight and review dry weight!

Pain on cannulation of arterio-venous fistulae

In many patients, the skin at venepuncture site has been rendered insensitive by repeated venepuncture and anaesthesia is not required. There is little benefit from injection of local anaesthetics. Placement of Emla cream at proposed needle entry sites for 60 minutes before inserting the needle may reduce the discomfort.

Persistent bleeding from fistula exit site

Firm pressure with a gloved finger applied to a gauze swab over the site will usually suffice. If this fails fill the cap of a container (2 cm diameter) fully with cotton wool and place (cotton wool down) over the site. Tape firmly in place with bandage, twisting bandage each time it crosses the cap.

Restless leg syndrome

A common problem in dialysis patients and others with advanced CRI. A variety of pharmacological regimens have been tried with some success, including:

Clonazepam (0.25 mg starting dose, maximal daily dose 2 mg one hour before bedtime) may be effective with a low risk of adverse effects.

Diazepam 2 mg once a day PO is useful in mild cases.

Levodopa in a titrated dose of 50 to 150 mg at bedtime is recommended for elderly patients.

Gabapentin 300 mg od PO; cr.cl. <15 ml/min 100 mg od PO; and HD patients 200 mg after dialysis (Thorp et al; 2001).

Treatment of anemia with erythropoietin or treatment of iron deficiency with iron may result in the improvement of symptoms of restless leg syndrome.

Seizures on haemodialysis

Stop haemodialysis.
Diazepam 10–20 mg by IV injection at a rate of 0.5 ml (2.5 mg) per 30 seconds.
Clonazepam 1 mg in1 ml solution over 30 seconds IV
Check urgent blood sugar: if hypoglycemia suspected inject 50 ml of 50% glucose IV.

Tuberculosis treatment

With the increase of multidrug-resistant strains therapy should include a minimum of four antituberculous drugs until sensitivities are known.
Initial therapy (2 months):
Isoniazid (INH)
Rifampicin
Pyrazinamide
Ethambutol
Of these, at least two drugs should be continued for an additional 4–10 months according to sensitivity results. Therapy should last for a

total of 12 months for pulmonary TB and for 18 months for extrapulmonary TB.

Vascular access

Permanent vascular access is a-v fistula or PTFE grafts. A-V fistula should be the first option.

Vascular access should be considered at least 3–4 months before the scheduled beginning of dialysis, when GFR is <25 mL/min, or serum creatinine >4 mg/dL.

PTFE graft is immediately available for puncture; a-v fistula is usually ready for puncture after 3–4 months. In any case, do not puncture a-v fistula sooner than 10 days after operation.

Vitamin supplementation in dialysis patients

- vitamin C 100 mg od PO
- folic acid 1 mg od
- vitamin E 200 mg PO od
- vitamin B6 10–50 mg od PO
- avoid vitamin-A containing multivitamin preparations as plasma concentration of vitamin A and retinol binding proteins is increased in renal insufficiency.

HEPATITIS B

Prevention and immunization best policy. If HBV positive dialyze in isolation.

Lamivudine can be used as primary therapy in patients with chronic HBV infection who have active virus replication (serum HBV DNA positive by non-PCR assay, HBeAg positive or negative) and active liver disease (elevated serum ALT >two times normal and evidence of moderate/severe chronic hepatitis on liver biopsy)

Lamivudine should be administered orally in doses of 100 mg/day PO for one year. Dose reduction is necessary in patients with renal insufficiency (creatinine clearance <50 mL/min).

The optimal duration of therapy is uncertain. In patients with HBeAg positive chronic hepatitis B, the end-point of treatment is HBeAg seroconversion. It is reasonable to check HBV DNA levels every three months to monitor for antiviral response and breakthrough infection, and to check HBeAg and HBeAb at 9 and 12 months to assess for HBeAg seroconversion. Based upon data that are currently available, discontinuation of Lamivudine after one year can be considered in patients who have sustained HBeAg seroconversion.

Interferon alpha 3 million u x3/week is also approved for treatment of patients with aminotransferase levels > 2x elevated, HBeAg +ve and who have chronic hepatitis on biopsy.

HEPATITIS C

Treatment of chronic hepatitis C consists of interferon alfa (standard or pegylated) alone or in combination with ribavirin: interferon alfa (alfa 2a or 2b) 3 million units SC three times weekly for 24 weeks and then 48 weeks. Steroid therapy may be used in interferon-alfa resistant cases.

Relapse after interferon monotherapy: patients who relapse after an initial response to interferon monotherapy should receive for 24 or 48 weeks combination therapy interferon alfa with ribavirin PO (patient <75 kg: 600 mg mane, 400 mg nocte; patient > 75 kg: 600 mg bd).

Better response to therapy is with combination of ribavirin and pegylated interferon alfa 2-b for 48 weeks. The initial dose is pegylated interferon alpha 2-b 1 microgram/kg/week for 12 weeks plus ribavirin 1000–1200 mg/d, followed by pegylated interferon alpha 2-b 1.5 microgram/kg/week for 36 weeks plus ribavirin 800 mg/d. The other option is pegylated interferon alfa 2-a 180 micrograms/week.

Patients should be informed of the potential adverse effects of interferon and ribavirin. The main adverse events related to interferon are depression, hypothyoidism, influenza-like symptoms and alopecia. The main adverse events related to ribavirin are anemia and teratogenicity. Therefore absolute contraindication to ribavirin is pregnancy.

Acetaminophen 600 mg PO can be given concomitantly with interferon to prevent flu-like symptoms. The important side-effects of interferon therapy are thrombocytopaenia and neutropaenia. The dose of interferon should be reduced, or discontinued if neutrophil count <750 cells/mm^3.

Treatment with interferon-alfa is recommended for patients on hemodialysis with active hepatitis on liver biopsy and hepatitis C infected dialysis patients who are candidates for renal transplantation. A regimen of three million units of interferon-alfa three times per week following each HD session for 6 to 12 months (if tolerated) appears to be safe and effective in inducing biochemical and virological responses. The dose of interferon in chronic renal insufficiency can be reduced to 1.5-million x3/wk.

Ribavirin is contraindicated in women who are or can become pregnant and also in patients with CRF.

The immunostimulant effects of interferon alfa can result in enhanced allograft rejection when interferon alfa is used in the transplant recipient with hepatitis C, therefore renal transplant is a contraindication to treatment with interferon.

Ribavirin was not associated with any detrimental side effects on graft function but its use is limited to patients with a creatinine clearance above 50 mL/min.

HEPATO-RENAL SYNDROME

Avoid drugs and procedures that may adversely affect the patient with liver disease: NSAID, lactulose (hypovolaemia), aminoglycosides, vigorous diuresis, and large volume paracentesis. Treat infection early.

Therapeutic options with limited success include:

- Terlipressin 2 mg bolus IV followed by 1–2 mg every 4–6 hours
- Infusion of 20% human albumin 1g/kg first day, followed by 20–40 g daily for 5–15 days
- Dopamine 1–5 µg/kg/min IV infusion (controversial).
- Paracentesis of ascites fluid with substitution of proteins with human albumin (infuse 6–8 g albumin for every litre of fluid removed)
- Continuous arteriovenous or venovenous haemofiltration with bicarbonate (instead of lactate) as the buffer for replacement fluid can be used as a holding measure in resistant cases, for example whilst awaiting urgent liver transplantation.

Hepato-renal syndrome is invariably fatal unless there is a prospect of hepatic recovery or transplantation.

HICCUPS

Try chlorpromazine 25 mg tds PO.
Or haloperidol 1.5 mg up to three times daily
Sometimes ingestion of ice cream or similar cold (frozen) product may help.

HYPERCALCAEMIA

Treat the underlying cause.
Usual cause for hypercalcaemia in patient on dialysis is iatrogenic; therefore reduce or stop alfacalcidol or calcitriol, change from calcium based phosphate binders to Sevelamer (Renagel).
Replace water and electrolyte deficit as follows:
- mild hypercalcemia (serum calcium <12 mg/dL): oral hydration, increase salt intake;
- moderate hypercalcemia (serum calcium 12.0–13.5 mg/dL) and severe hypercalcemia (serum calcium >13.5 mg/dL): rehydrate with isotonic saline (up to 3–4 L/24 hours); diuretic (Frusemide 40 mg bd IV) after rehydration; hemodialysis with low calcium concentrate in the dialysate (not calcium free dialysate) and/or antiresorptive therapy with bisphosphonates. Bisphosphonates: disodium pamidronate 30 mg in 250 ml isotonic saline infused IV over 2–4 hours (single dose) for serum calcium <3 mmol/L; 60 mg of sodium pamidronate if serum calcium 3 – 3.4 mmol/L and 90 mg sodium pamidronate in divided doses for serum calcium > 3.4 mmol/L. Reduce the dose by 50% for renal failure. Pamidronate IV once in 3–4 weeks.

Steroids are effective in the treatment of hypercalcaemia in sarcoidosis.

HYPERHOMOCYSTEINAEMIA

Folic acid 5 mg three times/week plus Vit B1, B6 and B12 (if patient is on haemodialysis, give doses post-haemodialysis).

HYPERKALAEMIA

Reduce dietary intake of potassium. Stop potassium supplements, potassium-retaining diuretics (spironolactone, amiloride), ACEI and AIIRA.

ECG changes reflect extreme urgency: the first symptom of hyperkalaemia can be sudden death! Each of the following is emergency treatments that buy some time, but unless the underlying cause is reversed the hyperkalaemia will recur.

- 10 ml 10% calcium gluconate IV slowly over 5 minutes, check ECG in 15 minutes and if still abnormal, repeat once or twice, total dose up to 40 ml. Alternatively 10 mL of 10% Calcium chloride IV over 5 minutes. This measure protects the heart against the consequences of hyperkalaemia but does not lower serum potassium.
- 50 ml 50% glucose + 10 Units soluble Insulin IV over 30 minutes. Check blood sugar after few minutes but hypoglycaemia is uncommon with this regimen. This treatment drives potassium into cells and transiently lowers serum potassium. Can be repeated but each treatment may only last 20–30 minutes and simply buys time for definitive measures to be applied to the underlying cause.
- in the setting of chronic hyperkalemia polystyrene sulphonate resin (Kayexalate/Calcium resonium/Resonium A) 10–15 g in 100 mL of water PO up to four times/day PO or alternatively PR). Prescribe a laxative or irrigation to remove resin from colon. Polystyrene sulphonate resin can be given per rectum as enema 30 g in methylcellulose solution. It should be retained in rectum for 30–60 min. Cleansing enema should be given afterwards to prevent drug retention in colon and to reduce the risk of intestinal necrosis.
- if hyperkalemia is associated with severe metabolic acidosis (arterial blood pH <7.2) give 1 ampule (45 mEq) of 7.5% sodium bicarbonate solution IV slowly over 5 minutes or 50 ml 8.4% Sodium bicarbonate IV over 30 minutes.
- albuterol nebulizer 10–20 mg over 10 minutes is similar in efficacy to dextrose + insulin.

- loop (frusemide 20–40 mg od PO/IV) or thiazide diuretics transiently reduce plasma potassium concentration, specially in conditions with low urine output (and low potassium excretion)
- if conservative measures are ineffective or insufficient, last option is dialysis. Removal of potassium is much faster with haemodialysis than with haemofiltration or peritoneal dialysis. Low potassium bath should be used (i.e. 1 mEq/L).

HYPERNATRAEMIA
(Serum sodium > 150 mEq/L)

Correct extracellular volume depletion with isotonic saline, followed by correction of hypernatraemia with 5% dextrose + 1/2 isotonic saline.

If hypernatraemia is associated with extracellular volume expansion, diuretic (frusemide) can be used to treat hypernatraemia. Patients in renal failure with hypervolaemia and hypernatraemia need dialysis for correction of these abnormalities.

Patient with euvolaemic hypernatraemia can be treated primarily with water (5% dextrose). For 82 kg patient with serum sodium concentration of 152 mEq/L, the amount of water could be calculated according to the formula:

Total body water = body weight x 60%
Total body water = 82 x 0.6 = 49.2
Actual plasma sodium/desired plasma sodium x total body water = 152/142 x 49.2 = 52.66 L. Therefore this patient needs (52.66–49.2 = 3.46) liters of water (D5%) to correct hypernatraemia. This fluid can be given orally or parenterally.

HYPERPROLACTINAEMIA

Hyperprolactinaemia is common in patients with renal failure and usually asymptomatic. If treatment is indicated, bromocriptine can be given, 1–1.25 mg PO at bedtime, increasing by 500 µg weekly to usual dose of 2.5 mg twice daily. Often causes nausea.

If pituitary tumour > 10 mm diameter and if bromocriptine therapy is ineffective or not tolerated, then surgery (usually transphenoidal approach) is indicated.

HYPERTENSION

(See Chronic Renal Insufficiency, Diabetes mellitus, Renal Transplant, Pregnancy)

Target blood pressure of <130/85 in all patients with renal disease. Target blood pressure of <125/75 in patients with urinary protein excretion >1g/d.

Patients with renal diseases or functioning renal transplant who are not on dialysis frequently require multiple antihypertensive medications.

ACEI are the first line antihypertensive drugs in patients with nephropathies, proteinuria, especially diabetic nephropathy in all stages (microalbuminuria, proteinuria, nephrotic range proteinuria and even in renal insufficiency). Unfortunately, they are not too efficient in polycystic kidney disease. There are no significant differences between various drugs in this class; they are all once daily and per os:

Enalapril 2.5, 5, 10 and 20 mg od PO
Lisinopril 2.5, 5, 10 and 20 mg od PO
Perindopril 2 and 4 mg od PO
Ramipril 1.25, 2.5, 5 and 10 mg od PO
Captopril 6.25 mg bd PO and increase to 12.5 – 25 – 50 mg bd PO

If the patient does not tolerate ACEI (especially due to cough, a common adverse effect) the alternative with comparable effects (but not causing cough) is an Angiotensin II receptor antagonist (AIIRA):

Candesartan 2, 4, 8, 16 mg od PO
Irbesartan 150, 300 mg od PO
Losartan 25–50 mg od PO
Valsartan 40–80 mg od PO

Serum concentrations of potassium and creatinine should be checked in all patients seven days after the initiation of treatment with ACEI or AIIRA. It is common to notice a reduction in glomerular filtration rate (5–15%) within 1–4 weeks of initiation of therapy with these drugs. This reduction of GFR is usually reversible. However, if the patient has an acute rise of serum creatinine of more than 30%–50%, the possibility of renal artery stenosis should be explored and ACEI/AIIRA stopped. Hyperkalaemia is also a side effect of

ACEI/AIIRA, combination with loop diuretics can at least partly control it.

Diuretic therapy potentates the antihypertensive effects of most other antihypertensive drugs. For this reason they should be added as a second-step agent if blood pressure is inadequately controlled with any other drug chosen as a first-line agent.

Bendrofluazide 2.5 and 5 mg, od PO in the morning or on alternate days
Hydrochlorothiazide 12.5–25 mg od PO.
Chlorthalidone 25–50 mg od (in the morning) PO.
Metolazone 5 mg od
Thiazide diuretics have limited effect in renal insufficiency (serum creatinine >200 μmol/l).
Loop diuretics (frusemide 20 and 40 mg PO or 20–50 mg IV; or slow IV infusion 250 mg over 1 hour) could be used in renal insufficiency, if needed they may be combined with thiazides, and in refractory cases with metolazone.

Potassium sparing diuretics should only be used with extreme caution in renal insufficiency (high risk of hyperkalaemia).

Long acting Calcium channel blockers (CCB):

Dihydropyridine CCB:
Amlodipine 5–10 mg OD
Nifedipine (Adalat LA 20, 30, 60 mg tbl, dose 20 mg OD and increase if necessary, max. 90 mg daily; Adalat SR 10 and 20 mg OD).

Non-dihydropyridine CCB:
Verapamil 240–480 mg daily in 2–3 divided doses
Diltiazem SR90, 120, 180 mg OD, Diltiazem XL 120, 180 and 240 mg OD.

Beta-blockers:
Atenolol 25–100 mg od PO
Bisoprolol 5–10 mg od PO

Alpha blocker:
Doxazosin is the most often used drug in this class of antihypertensive drugs. The starting dose is 1 mg od PO (at bedtime), increase if needed to 2 mg od PO thereafter to 4 mg od if necessary; maximum dose 16 mg od PO. Alpha-blockers may be

used in combination with other classes of anti-hypertensive drugs, but not as first line therapy.

Direct vasodilatators:
Minoxidil 2.5 mg (elderly patients) or 5 mg daily in 1–2 doses PO. Minoxidil causes marked renal salt and water retention; therefore patients treated with this drug usually require additional treatment with a potent loop diuretic.
Hydralazine 25 mg bd PO, increase to 50 mg bd PO if necessary

Combination of anti-hypertensive drugs:
In general therapy should start with a single drug. If blood pressure is not optimally controlled with one drug, various combinations of drugs may be effective. In these combinations even the lower doses of individual components may be used.

ACEI + diuretic; ACEI + CCB; CCB + diuretic; CCB + beta-blocker; beta-blocker + diuretic. As third line drug alpha-blocker can be added.

Most antihypertensive drugs can be given on a once-daily basis, and this should be the goal to improve patient compliance.

Algorithm for achieving target blood pressure in patients with renal disease

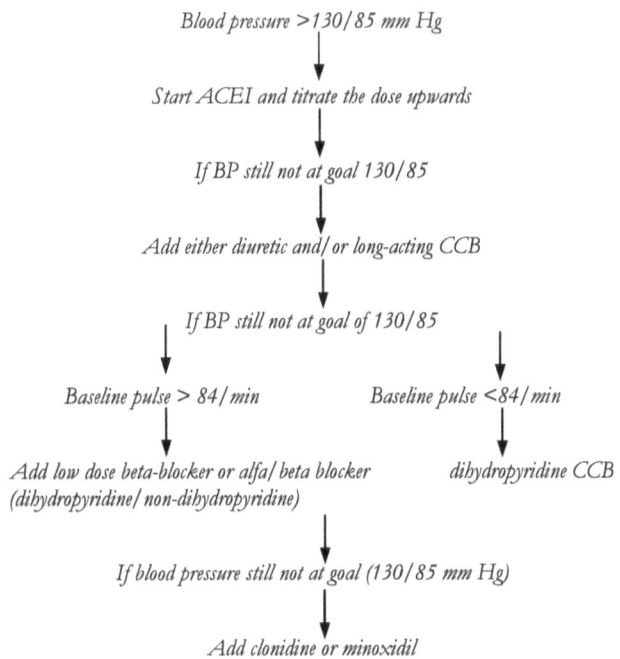

Hypertensive urgency (diastolic BP >120 mmHg without acute end-organ damage):

Instead of lowering the blood pressure within hours, the blood pressure can gradually be lowered over days to weeks if there is no immediate danger of end-organ damage. At present, there is no data indicating that acute reduction is better than gradual reduction.

Whether lowered within 24 hours or within a week, oral agents should be the first line of therapy for hypertensive urgency. The most commonly used oral agents include:
- Clonidine 0.1–0.2 mg up to three times daily PO or
- Labetalol 100 mg bd PO, increase at intervals of 14 days to usual dose of 200 mg twice daily. By IV injection 50 mg over at least 1 minute, repeat after 5 minutes if necessary, max. 200 mg or

- Minoxidil 2,5–5 mg bd PO

Although these are commonly used, it makes sense to initiate a medication that will be indicated for long-term use. Since the cause of hypertensive urgency is frequently secondary to nonadherence to previously prescribed antihypertensive therapy (calcium channel blockers or ACEI/AIIRA), simply reinitiating the same medicines often works well. It is important to continue to monitor the patient and have him/her return within 1–2 weeks to ensure that the blood pressure is improving and that there are no further complications of uncontrolled hypertension.

Hypertensive emergency:

In patients with neurological presentations avoid the use of antihypertensive drugs that may impair mental status (clonidine, methyldopa).

- Treat diastolic BP greater than 140 mm Hg with sodium nitroprusside 0.3 μg/kg/min as IV infusion. The recommended starting dose of Nitroprusside is 0.25 to 0.5 μg/kg per minute. This can be increased as necessary to a maximum dose of 8 to 10 μg/kg per minute; maximum doses of 10 μg/kg per minute should never be given for more than 10 minutes. The use of Nitroprusside is the treatment of choice for patients requiring parenteral therapy. It is short acting. Infusion set should be wrapped in foil since drug is unstable when exposed to light.
- Oral antihypertensive agents should be initiated as soon as possible to minimize the duration of parenteral therapy. The Nitroprusside infusion can be weaned as the oral agents become effective. Nitroprusside should not be given to pregnant women.
- Second choice is labetalol. It can be used successfully in preeclamptic patients. It can be given as an intravenous bolus or infusion. The bolus dose is 20 mg IV over 2 minute; repeat after 5 minutes if necessary, max. 200 mg. For IV infusion make a solution of 1 mg/ml by diluting the contents of two ampoules (200 mg) to 200 ml with 5% dextrose. Give by IV infusion 0.5–2 mg/min until satisfactory response.

- In patients with cardiovascular presentations (left ventricular failure and hypertension) IV nitroglycerin and nitroprusside are effective therapies. The initial dose of nitroglycerin is 5 μg/min, which can be increased as necessary to a maximum of 100 μg/min.
- Hydralazine is drug of choice in eclampsia, but should be avoided in unstable angina, myocardial infarction or aortic dissection. The initial dose given as an intravenous bolus is 5–10 mg diluted with 10 ml isotonic saline, may be repeated after 20–30 minutes, with the maximum dose being 20 mg. Hydralazine can be given by intravenous infusion, initially 200–300 μg/min, maintenance usually 50–150 μg/min.
- Nicardipine 5–15 mg/hr IV is one of a few dihydropyridine CCB currently used to treat hypertension, it does not usually produce a sudden fall in BP.

One should aim for a gradual reduction of blood pressure to normotensive levels over a few days to a week. Oral antihypertensive drugs should be initiated as soon as possible to minimize the duration of parenteral therapy.

HYPOCALCAEMIA

Supplement calcium orally as calcium acetate, calcium citrate or calcium carbonate between meals or overnight.

In an emergency: 10% Calcium gluconate 10 ml amp slow IV injection over 20 min followed (if needed) by IV infusion 10% Calcium gluconate 50 ml in 500 ml 5% Dextrose over 8 hours.

In hypoparathyroidism, and especially immediately post-parathyroidectomy, in addition to IV calcium give Alfacalcidol 0.25–5 micrograms/d PO.

Correct hypomagnesaemia if associated with hypocalcaemia.

In patients with hypercalciuria give spironolactone or amiloride or hydrochlorothiazide to reduce urinary loss of calcium.

HYPOKALAEMIA

Correct the underlying cause (diarrhoea, vomiting, diuretics, and inadequate intake). In patients with impaired renal function, give potassium supplements and/or potassium-sparing diuretics with great caution!

Mild – moderate (K > 2.5 mmol/L): give potassium salt 60–80 mmol/d preferably orally. Tablets: Sando-K 12 mmol potassium (2 tbl bd PO) or Slow-K 8 mmol/tbl, Syrup (Kay-Cee-L) 1 mmol/mL.

If hypokalemia is severe (K < 2.5 mmol/L): give 120–160 mmol/d of potassium salt IV, but maximum replacement 20 mmol/h in a solution that contains maximum potassium of 40 mmol/L.

Restrict water intake to as little as 500 mL/d!

For prevention of hypokalemia use potassium chloride 2–4 g (25–50 mmol) daily PO.

HYPONATRAEMIA (plasma sodium <135 mEq/L)

Search and treat underlying disorder (salt loss, adrenal insufficiency). Ideally, allow spontaneous correction or use oral supplements.
In an emergency (eg convulsions) can treat with combination of hypertonic saline (3%) IV infusion at a rate 1–2 ml/kg/h (1.0 – 1.5 mEq/L/h) and a loop diuretic (Frusemide 40 mg) until convulsions subside. Do not exceed a correction rate of 1.5 mEq/h. Do not increase serum concentration of sodium by more than 10% (12–15 mEq/d) as full correction done too fast is potentially harmful (pontine myelinolysis)
Do not increase serum sodium by more than 15 mEq/L per 24 h. Restrict water intake to as little as 500 ml/d.

INFLUENZA

Zanamavir 10 mg BD for 5 days. Indicated to treat influenza in high-risk patients, especially elderly. Take within 48 hours after the onset of symptoms or when influenza is epidemic in the community.

INSOMNIA

(See Restless legs syndrome)

Patients with insomnia frequently require long-term pharmacological management.

Pharmacological therapy — Hypnotic medications should generally not be the treatment of first choice for chronic insomnia. Hypnotic medications are contraindicated in pregnancy; these drugs should be used judiciously in patients with renal disease. As a first choice use zopiclone (7.5 mg at bed time) or zolpidem (5 mg at bed time), and if this is not effective, try temazepam (10 mg at bed time). Ask patients to use them sparingly e.g. once or twice/week

INOTROPES

Choice of inotropic/vasopressor therapy depends on the medical condition causing hypotension. In cardiogenic shock due to myocardial infarction the first choice agent depends on the BP: if >90mmHg = dobutamine; if BP 80–90 mmHg = dopamine; and if BP <80 mmHg = noradrenaline.
In septic shock noradrenaline is the first coice and dobutamine should be added if cardiac output is low.

Dopamine as IV infusion: 2–5 µg/kg/min (renal dose); 10 µg/kg/min (vasopressor dose); may be increased by 1–4 µg/kg/min at 10– to 30–minute intervals and titrate up to 20 µg/kg/min until optimal response is obtained. If dosage >20 µg/kg/min are needed, a more direct-acting pressor may be more beneficial (i.e. adrenaline, noradrenaline).

Noradrenaline IV infusion; initiate at 4 µg/min and titrate to desired response; 8 – 12 µg/min is usual range. Dosing range 0.05– 30 µg/min.

Dobutamine IV infusion 2.5–15 µg/kg/min, maximum 40 µg/kg/min, titrate to desired response.

All the inotropes/vasopressors (with the exception of dobutamine) should be administered via a central line.

The dose (µg/kg/min) as infusion volume (mL/hour), adjusted to patient's weight (kg) can be found in accompanying leaflet or published tables.

INTERSTITIAL NEPHRITIS

Stop the incriminated drug (if drug related) or treat underlying infection.
Corticosteroids: prednisolone 1 mg/kg/day, but for only limited time e.g. 6–8 weeks.

If ARF is severe (creatinine >700 μmol/L) pulse Methylprednisolone 1 g daily IV for three consecutive days may be used.
When improvement of renal function is achieved, gradually reduce steroid dose. Total duration of steroid therapy 2–3 months.

IV IMMUNOGLOBULINS

0.4 g/kg/day for 5 days on a monthly basis. Antihistamines may be useful as pre-treatment if allergic phenomena occur. Reversible decline in renal function may be seen in patients with renal impairment, diabetes mellitus, volume depletion, and older age: this may be due to renal tubular toxicity of the diluent and varies from preparation to preparation. Glycine based diluent IVIG's are safe, while sucrose-based IVIG's put patient at risk to develop acute renal failure. Sucrose-based IVIG should be given slowly, the patient shoud be well hydrated and not on diuretic.

LEGIONELLA INFECTION

Azithromycin 500 mg od PO for three days
Or
Erythromycin 250–500 mg qds IV first week, afterwards 250–500 mg qds PO for three weeks.

LEPTOSPIROSIS

Benzylpenicillin (Penicillin G) 2.4 g qds IM or slow IV injection or infusion
Or Amoxicillin 500 mg qds PO
Or Doxycycline 100 mg bd PO

MENINGITIS

- Benzylpenicillin 2.4 g slow IV every 4 hours or
- Cefotaxime (if penicillin allergic) 2–4 g tds IV or
- Ceftriaxone 2 g bd IV

MESNA

Mesna reacts with acrolein, a toxic metabolite of cyclophosphamide which can cause haemorrhagic cystitis. Mesna is used to protect the urinary bladder when high dose of intravenous cyclophosphamide are given. Mesna commonly causes adverse reactions itself including headache, rash, nausea and vomiting, effects often also associated with cyclophosphamide. If in doubt, it is reasonable to omit mesna to test whether cyclophosphamide itself is tolerated. In patients with well-preserved excretory renal function, an alternative is to fluid load the patient (orally or intravenously) and encourage frequent bladder emptying.

Oral MESNA has 50% the bioavailability of intravenous and takes about 2 hours to be excreted into the urine. Therefore a regimen for the use of Mesna is:

Time 0: give cyclophosphamide ("C") with Mesna (20% of "C") mg in 500 ml of 0.9% sodium chloride over 1 hour. This is made in Pharmacy (24 hours notice is needed).

Time 0 + 2 hrs: Give Mesna (40% of "C") mg PO

Time 0 + 6 hrs: Give Mesna (40% of "C") mg PO

It is preferable to give more rather than less Mesna so one could broadly group doses as follows:

Cyclophosphamide dose	>500 mg	>500 mg–1 g	1.1–1.5 g
MESNA IV	100 mg	200 mg	300 mg
MESNA PO	200 mg	400 mg	600 mg

Tablets come as 400 mg and 600 mg. For 200 mg dose give half of a 400 mg tablet.

METHANOL INTOXICATION

(See Ethylene glycol intoxication)

MINOR SURGICAL AND DENTAL PROCEDURES (in CRF and renal transplant patients)

Antibiotics before surgical procedures (dental procedures, endoscopies, cystoscopy, etc): Amoxicillin 3 g sachet PO one hour before intervention (one dose). If patient is allergic to penicillin, give Erythromycin 1 g orally before intervention, or Clarithromycin 500 mg one dose PO/IV Or
Ampicillin 2 g IM/IV 30 min before the procedure (one dose) Or Vancomycin 1 g od IV before the intervention (one dose).

MIXED CRYOGLOBULINAEMIA

Prior to discovery of the association with HCV, both prednisolone and cytotoxic drugs were often used as therapy in patients with slowly progressive disease. However, immunosuppressive therapy may increase hepatitis C virus replication and may worsen the viral infection.

Aggressive therapy in idiopathic mixed cryoglobulinaemia is primarily reserved for patients with acute disease; it includes plasmapheresis to remove the circulating cryoglobulins and pulses of IV methylprednisolone:

- Plasmapheresis prescription: exchange one plasma volume (4L) every other day for two to three weeks. Replacement fluid: five percent albumin, which must be warmed to prevent precipitation of circulating cryoglobulins.
- Pulses of 1000 mg IV methylprednisolone daily for three days followed by conventional oral prednisolone and cyclophosphamide to prevent new antibody formation.

If cryoglobulinaemia is a manifestation of chronic HCV infection, then antiviral treatment with interferon alfa (preferably pegylated interferon) alone or in combination with ribavirin should be considered. Ribavirin is not recommended for patients with a creatinine clearance below 50 mL/min. Such individuals should be treated with interferon alfa alone.

Therapy should be delayed for two to four months in patients with severe disease who are initially treated with plasmapheresis and immunosuppressive therapy.

Patients who progress to end-stage renal disease can be treated with dialysis or renal transplantation. Survival on either hemodialysis or peritoneal dialysis is similar to that in patients with other renal diseases, although sick patients have a higher early mortality rate.

Renal transplantation has been successfully performed in mixed cryoglobulinaemia.

NASAL SCREENING FOR DIALYSIS PATIENTS

Nasal carriage of Staphylococcus aureus increases the risk of invasive staphylococcal infections, dialysis catheter infections etc. Nasal carriage can be eradicated by treatment with mupirocin cream (see below). We recommend regular screening of dialysis patients according to the following protocol.

Anterior nasal swabs should be taken from each nostril at monthly intervals in hospital-based patients (who are at highest risk) and at three monthly intervals in community-based patients. Patients with positive swabs should be treated with a 5 day course of mupirocin cream (2% Bactroban cream), applied to each nostril three times daily. All patients should be re-screened a month later and the course of mupirocin repeated for any remaining positives.

NAUSEA AND VOMITING

Management of nausea and vomiting should include:
- Recognition and correction of any cases such as recognition and replacement of any depleted fluid, electrolyte, as well as identification and correction of acid–base and metabolic disturbances.
- Identification, wherever possible, of the underlying cause (vomiting of central origin; gastrointestinal obstruction; pseudoobstruction; gastrointestinal dysmotility and gastroparesis; functional and psychogenic vomiting; drug toxicity eg digoxin), followed by appropriate therapy
- Where necessary, therapeutic strategies to suppress or eliminate symptoms.

Symptomatic therapy should be based on symptom severity and clinical context.

Thus mild nausea and uncomplicated vomiting may be treated empirically with oral antiemetics:

Metoclopramide 10 mg od-tds PO/IM/IV (avoid in severe renal failure);

Domperidone 10 mg tds PO;

Ondansetron 8 mg bd PO or IM/IV;

Haloperidol 0.5–2 mg PO.

Severe intractable episodes require parenteral administration of such agents as Chlorpromazine hydrochloride 25–50 mg IM; Haloperidol 2–10 mg IM/IV.

The prevention and treatment of both acute cancer chemotherapy-related and postoperative nausea and vomiting have come to be based largely on the use of Granisetron 1–2 mg od-bd PO or 1 mg IV diluted in 5 ml in D5% or isotonic saline or Ondansetron 8 mg bd PO or IM/IV.

The commonest situation that Nephrologists encounter nausea and vomiting is renal failure, in which case dialyse!

NEPHROTIC SYNDROME

Bed rest (stimulate diuresis). However, in view of increased thrombotic risk this should be accompanied by anti-thrombotic precautions. Immersion in water (eg a swimming pool) can help to mobilise oedema.
Restrict salt. Restrict fluid intake to 1–1.5 L/day.
Monitor blood pressure and treat hypertension preferably with ACEI or AIIRA. Blood pressure control should be targeted to values <130/80 mm Hg. ACEI and AIIRA have antiproteinuric effect and can be given to normotensive patients. The dose of these drugs should be titrated against urinary protein excretion apart from their antihypertensive action. Starting doses (example): Captopril 12.5 mg bd PO or Enalapril 2.5 mg od PO or Losartan 25 mg od PO.
Combined therapy ACEI + AIIRA have a stronger antiproteinuric effect than single therapy with a maximal dose of an ACEI or an AIIRA.

Diuretics: loop diuretic (Frusemide 40–80 mg od orally, if no effect increase the dose to 120 mg – 160 mg orally, or 40–80–120–250 mg IV and finally, if needed 10–40 mg/hour as constant IV infusion). If no response, consider combination of diuretic (Frusemide + Metolazone 5 mg od orally).
In patients with severe hypoalbuminaemia coadministration of frusemide with albumin is significantly more effective than frusemide alone (60 mg of IV frusemide + 200 ml of 20% solution of albumin). Statin if patient has hyperlipidaemia.

Anticoagulate (Warfarin) if prolonged treatment or high risk of DVT/PE/Renal vein thrombosis (especially with membranous nephropathy).

NEUTROPAENIC PATIENTS (pyrexia episodes)

NB doses of many of drugs mentioned here need modification in patients with impaired renal function (see individual drugs).

<u>With normal renal function:</u>

Oral prophylaxis
Ciprofloxacin 250 mg po BD
Fluconazole 100 mg od PO loading dose, afterwards 50 mg od PO every other day (three times per week)
Acyclovir 200 mg tds PO
Co-trimoxazole 480–960 mg/d every other day (three times/week)

First line antibiotics for pyrexial episodes:

Piperacillin up to 4 g tds IV(if the patient is allergic to piperacillin, use ceftazidime 2 g tds)
Gentamicin up to 7 mg/kg in 100 ml normal saline IV or 5% dextrose over 1 hour (check blood level before next dose, trough level should be < 2 mg/L)
Vancomycin 1 g in 100 ml isotonic saline slow IV infusion over 100 min. (check blood level before next dose, pre-dose trough level should be <10 mg/L)
If pelvic/rectal/oral symptoms add metronidazole 400 mg tds PO (if unable to take PO, give 500 mg tds IV)
Continue oral prophylaxis.

If temperature resolved (T < 37.5°C) continue oral prophylaxis if still neutropaenic (see above).

If cultures are negative: stop IV antibiotics once apyrexial for further 24 hours
If cultures positive: (a) gram positive bacteraemia, continue IV Vancomycin for a total of 7 days (check blood level), stop piperacillin and gentamicin.
Gram negative bacteraemia: continue i.v. Piperacillin or ceftazidime and gentamicin for a total of 10 days, if sensitive to gentamicin consider ciprofloxacin 500 mg bd PO as alternative. Stop vancomycin.

If mixed bacteraemia: (gram positive and gram negative): continue both vancomycin and piperacillin (or ceftazidime) and gentamicin and seek microbiology advice.

If fungal growth positive: consider anti-fungal therapy (watch LFTs): Itraconazole 200 mg daily and increase fluconazole to 400 mg daily) or Amphotericin 50 mg IV daily over 6 hours.

Lenograstim 19.2 million u/m^2 body surface area daily SC until neutrophil count in acceptable range. Body surface area = square root of [height (cm) X weight (kg)/3600].

NUTRITION (ORAL/TUBE FEEDING/PARENTERAL)

Oral supplements are indicated in patients in whom protein and calorie needs are not being met on a standard diet.

Naso-gastric tube feed is considered in patients with a functional gastrointestinal tract who are unable to maintain adequate protein and calorie nutrition with the use of diet or oral supplements and who are or may become malnourished. Ensure and Ensure Plus are often used. Ensure Plus ½ in normal saline up to 80 ml/hour, usually for 20 hours/day.

Nephro diluted 1 in 2 or 1 in 3 (undiluted preparation tends to cause diarrhoea).

Total parenteral nutrition is indicated in patients in whom the above is impossible or insufficient. A mixture of both essential and nonessential amino acids, fat and dextrose should provide a daily intake of 1.5 g/kg/d proteins and 30 – 35 kcal/kg/d. Proprietary infusions fluids for parenteral feeding such as Clinomet (Baxter) or KabiMix (Fresenius) are produced with different proportions of nitrogen (g/l), energy (kj/L) and electrolytes (mmol/L).

In ARF: 35 kcal/kg body weight/day, 1.2 g/kg protein, glucose: lipids = 70:30.In severely ill patients or patients in coma, total parenteral nutrition can be administered during haemodialysis.

PARACETAMOL (acetaminophen) POISONING

Although hepatic toxicity is the best recognised consequence of paracetamol (acetaminophen) overdose, acute renal failure (presumably due to acute tubular necrosis) is also seen, and can occur in the absence of major hepatic damage.

The mainstays of the therapy for paracetamol intoxication include gastrointestinal decontamination with activated charcoal and the administration of N-acetylcysteine.

Activated charcoal (AC) is the preferred method of gastrointestinal decontamination and is indicated for all patients who present within four hours of ingestion. AC should be administered as a single oral dose of one gram per kilogram body weight.

N-acetylcysteine (NAC) is the antidote of choice for the treatment of paracetamol poisoning. Serious hepatotoxicity is uncommon and death extremely rare, regardless of the initial serum paracetamol concentration, if NAC is administered within 8 to 10 hours following paracetamol.

NAC is indicated in the following situations:
- Patients with a serum paracetamol concentration above the "possible hepatic toxicity" line of the nomogram following an acute ingestion (British National Formulary 2002; p. 23);
- Patients with a single ingestion of greater than 10 – 15 g (20 – 30 tbl) or 150 mg/kg (or 7.5 g in an adult) by history and for whom results of a serum acetaminophen (paracetamol) concentration will not be available within 8 hours from the time of ingestion.
- Patients with an unknown time of ingestion and a serum acetaminophen concentration >10 mcg/mL.
- Patients with laboratory evidence of hepatotoxicity (from mildly elevated aminotransferase to fulminant hepatic failure) and a history of excessive acetaminophen ingestion.
- Patients who have ingested repeated excessive acetaminophen doses, have risk factors for acetaminophen-induced hepatotoxicity, and a serum acetaminophen concentration >10 mcg/mL.

NAC can be administered by either orally or IV. The 72–hour oral NAC regimen is more effective than the 20-hour intravenous regimen in reducing hepatotoxicity when treatment is delayed more than 10 hours.

72 h oral NAC treatment consists of a 140 mg/kg loading dose followed by 17 doses of 70 mg/kg every 4 hours (total dose 1330 mg/kg).

NAC is available as a 10 or 20 percent (10 or 20 g/100 mL) solution (Mucomyst). Nausea and vomiting are frequent side effects and antiemetics (See Nausea and Vomiting) should be administered in moderate to high doses.

A pyrogen-free NAC preparation can be administered by continuous intravenous infusion over a 20-hour period (total dose 300 mg/kg). Acetylcysteine within first 24 hours 150 mg/kg in 200 ml 5% glucose over 15 minutes followed by 50 mg/kg in 500 ml 5% glucose over 4 hours, followed by 100 mg/kg in 1000 ml 5% glucose over 16 hours.

Intravenous NAC is recommended for:
- Patients who cannot tolerate oral NAC due to vomiting and for whom further delay will result in decreased NAC efficacy (e.g., beyond 10 hours).
- Patients whose medical condition precludes enteral use of NAC (e.g., corrosive ingestion, gastrointestinal bleeding or obstruction).
- Patients with fulminant hepatic failure

All patients who develop acetaminophen-induced hepatic failure should be transferred to a centre specialized in the care of such patients and capable of performing liver transplantation

PEPTIC ULCER AND ERADICATION OF HELICOBACTER PYLORI

One week therapy with:
Omeprazole 20 mg bd PO, then 20 mg od PO for 5 weeks.
Plus
Amoxicillin 1 g bd PO
Plus
Clarithromycin 500 mg bd PO

Alternative regimen that does not include Clarithromycin:
Omeprazole 20 mg po bd PO (or Lansoprazole 30 mg po bd PO)
Plus
Metronidazole 400 mg bd PO

plus
Amoxicillin 1 g bd PO

PERIOPERATIVE MANAGEMENT (of patients with CRF/renal replacement)

Pre-Op Evaluation of patients with Renal Failure

For patients with GFR > 50 ml/min, no special precautions. For patients with GFR <50 ml/min, do physical examination, and obtain FBC, electrolytes, glucose, urea, creatinine, calcium, phosphorus, albumin, bicarbonate, coagulation status, ECG and CXR. Ensure dialysis if needed to achieve euvolaemia, normal serum K (optimal K pre-op is 4.0), blood pressure, blood pH, and serum Na. If bleeding risk for procedure high and if the patient is anaemic give a transfusion to Hct >30% or Hb >10 g/L. In those with pre-dialysis renal failure, set up IV fluids and maintain hydration.

If patient is already on dialysis, do pre-op HD session 12 – 24 hrs prior to surgical procedure to minimize risks of bleeding, fluid and electrolyte shifts, and haemodynamic instability. Do not remove too much fluid on dialysis as ESRD patients (especially patients with diabetes mellitus) are at risk for post induction hypotension, caused in part by autonomic instability. This can also be seen with spinal anaesthesia and post-op over-sedation.

If patient is on PD and there is minimal risk of hypoventilation or aspiration, the PD fluid can be drained and one-half the usual amount of fresh PD fluid replaced just prior to surgery. If patient at risk for hypoventilation or aspiration, peritoneal fluid should be drained just prior to the procedure. The PD catheter can be left in place if it is not in the line of surgical incision and if bacterial contamination of the peritoneum is neither present nor anticipated. Catheter should be filled with heparin-containing solution and capped. PD fluid and catheter should be manipulated only by personnel trained in peritoneal dialysis.

Remind the anaesthetist and surgeons to protect the dialysis access! Restrict fluid replacement to blood losses, insensible losses, and urine output if patient is clinically euvolaemic. If possible, avoid nephrotoxins (NSAIDs, IV contrast, and aminoglycosides). Even small amounts of residual renal function can be important for dialysis patients.

Monitor potassium levels and avoid potassium containing IV fluids, drugs which can effect peri-operative potassium levels (NSAIDs, beta blockers, heparin, and succinylcholine), and minimize blood products if possible. Remember to consider the full spectrum of medical management for hyperkalaemia including IV calcium, glucose and insulin, beta-agonists, and polystyrene sulphonate resins. Emergency dialysis may be needed if aggressive medical management is unsuccessful.

Intra-operative HD or haemofiltration have been performed during long or complicated cases to maintain metabolic and volume control.

Antibiotic prophylaxis for the haemodialysis access formation is controversial, but should be considered.

We do not advise routine perioperative use of antibiotics. However, in patients with diabetes mellitus and/or renal transplant and patients with a risk of bacterial infections, perioperative antibiotic prophylaxis may reduce the risk of wound infection.

Prophylactic antibiotics are given as one dose immediately before surgery. Many regimens and doses of antibiotics have been used. We prefer a first generation of cephalosporin given 30 minutes before incision Cephalozin 1.0 g IV/IM. The dose can be repeated if operation >4 hours.

Perioperative antibiotic prophylaxis to reduce the risk of wound infection with antibiotics directed against skin pathogens and urinary tract infection pathogens: Vancomycin 1 g slow IV over 100 min plus Cephalexin 250 mg qds PO or 500 mg bd PO. Other antibiotics that may be used include quinolones and beta-lactams. Antibiotics should be administered perioperatively and discontinued after 2–3 days after the operation to minimize the risk of resistant microorganism growth.

Antibiotic prophylaxis for dental procedures: Amoxicillin 3 g sachet 2–3 h before the procedure.

Antibiotic prophylaxis for intraabdominal operations (cholecystectomy, colorectal surgery etc):

- Augmentin 1.2 g IV at induction up to 2–3 further doses of 1.2 g may be given every 8 hours or

- Piperacillin 2.0 g IV one dose or Tazocin 2.25 g IV one dose

In high risk patients (prosthetic valves) Teicoplanin 400 mg IV initially three doses in interval of 12 hours then 200 mg od IV. Reconstitute initially with water for injection provided, infuse over 30 minutes.

Post-operative Recommendations

Monitor fluids, electrolytes, and haemodynamic status. PD can resume any time after non-abdominal surgery in most cases. After abdominal surgery, avoid restarting PD for 4–6 wks. When restarting PD, start with small volumes and frequent exchanges. HD tolerated better if not done during 24–48 hrs after surgery. Use heparin-free (or citrate) HD for the first few days post-op (may need to continue this for 1–2 wks post-op in some cases).

Postoperative pain can be managed with;

- Fentanyl 50 µg IV followed by 50 µg IV when required.
- opioids: morphine 5–10 mg SC/IM; Oramorph 5 mg PO every 4 hours: Pethidine (do not use in RI) 50 mg SC/IM; Diamorphine 5 mg SC/IM repeated every 4 hours if necessary.
- NSAID: Diclofenac 25 mg bd-tds; Ketoprofen 50 mg tds

Choose post-op pain medications carefully. Try to avoid NSAID (unless patient makes no urine), pethidine (active metabolites accumulate in renal impairment), morphine (ESRD patients sensitive to sedative effects and respiratory depressant effects), and codeine (similar to morphine; increase interval or decrease dose).

For patients who already have a permanent dialysis access, there is no research data to support prophylactic antibiotic use in patients undergoing procedures that may lead to bacteraemia, although many authors recommend it.

PLASMAPHERESIS (PE)

Avoid administration of ACEI before or during PE.

Administer 15 min before the procedure: 10 ml 10% calcium gluconate IV and 10 ml Chlorpheniramine (Piriton) IV and 100 ml Hydrocortisone IV
Ultrafiltration 500–1000 ml/hr

Total volume of Ultrafiltration/per session 4L
Frequency of PE: daily or on alternate days
Heparin: 5,000 u –10,000 u IV
If there is a risk of bleeding give FFP at the end of the procedure
Add 4 mEq of potassium to each liter of albumin solution given

PNEUMONIA

Community acquired pneumonia

Start treatment without delay and change from "blind" treatment to specific therapy after the results of serology and bacteriology became available.

Mild pneumonia:
- Clarithromycin 500 mg bd PO or
- Azithromycin 500 mg od for 7 days PO or
- Amoxicillin 500 mg tds PO or
- Doxycyclin 100 mg bd PO
- Levofloxacin/Moxifloxacin 500 mg od PO for 10 days

Moderate:
- Levofloxacin/Moxifloxacin 500 mg od PO or IV plus Clarithromycin 500 mg bd PO or
- Ceftriaxone 1 g od IV

Severe:
- Ceftriaxone 2 g IM/IV or
- Levofloxacin/Moxifloxacin 500 mg od IV plus Azithromycin 500 mg IV

Consider Pseudomonas aeruginosa infection that should be treated with:
- Ceftazidime 1 g tds IV or 2 g bd IV or
- Meropenem 500 mg tds IV or
- quinolones (Moxifloxacin 500 mg od or bd for 7–14 days)

PREGNANCY

Pregnancy is unusual in patients with more than moderate renal impairment and very rare in patients on dialysis. After successful renal transplantation, fertility is often restored. Pregnancy in patients with renal disease carries increased risks of pregnancy-associated hypertension, pre-term delivery, intra-uterine growth retardation and deterioration of maternal renal function.

Adult polycystic kidney disease (APCKD) and pregnancy

If family history is positive for subarachnoid hemorrhage; if patient was hypertensive during pregnancy, if MRI detected cerebral aneurysm previously – obstetrician and the patient may opt for Caesarian section (avoid natural labour).

Antiphospholipid syndrome and pregnancy

(See APS)

Pregnancy in women with CRI

In pregnant women with chronic renal disease, dialysis should be considered earlier than in non-pregnant patient. No evidence exists to support the superiority of one dialysis modality over another with respect to pregnancy outcome.

Haemodialysis sessions should be increased to 5–7 per week, with minimal heparinization and slow ultrafiltration to avoid dialysis hypotension and volume contraction.

If PD is used, decrease exchange volumes, and increase exchange frequencies.

Anaemia should be corrected with iron, folic acid, and erythropoietin.

Pre-eclampsia

Hospitalize!

Induce delivery if the gestation is near term and if there are signs of impending eclampsia: hyperreflexia, headaches, epigastric pain, blood pressure difficult to control, a rise in serum concentration of urea, creatinine, uric acid, transaminases.

Treatment of hypertension is described below (hydralazine, labetalol, calcium channel blockers). Avoid administration of diuretics since pre-eclampsia tends to be associated with low plasma volume.

Eclampsia convulsions

Magnesium sulphate is a drug of choice either as prophylactic therapy or for the treatment of convulsion. A loading dose of 4 g magnesium sulfate is infused over 15 minutes, followed by sustaining infusion of 1 to 2 g per hour aiming to achieve levels of 2 to 4 µmol/L.

Hyperemesis gravidarum

Promethazine hydrochloride (Phenergan) 25 mg at bedtime
Methylprednisolone 40 mg IV
Hydrocortisone 100 mg IV

Hypertension in pregnancy

Many of the recommendations regarding the appropriate treatment of hypertensive pregnant women are based on empirical data.

Lifestyle modifications, reduced physical activity, home blood pressure monitoring are all useful adjuncts to therapy.

Women with mild to moderate hypertension should be watched closely, warned about signs of early pre-eclampsia and delivered at 37 weeks of gestation.

The blood pressure normally decreases by the end of the first trimester and further in the second trimester. If the diastolic is between 90 and 100 mmHg in the first trimester, adjust the medications so they are appropriate for pregnancy; consider reducing the dosages of some of the medications, particular the diuretics. When diastolic BP is greater than 100 mmHg we would recommend treatment.

Specific antihypertensive drugs:

Alpha-methyldopa 250 mg bd or tds PO is a first-line antihypertensive agent in pregnancy.

Beta blockers: Labetalol 100 mg bd PO and increase after 14 days to 200 mg bd PO. It may be superior to some of the other beta-blockers because it preserves utero-placental blood flow to a greater degree than pure beta-blockers because of the alpha-blocking effects. Take with food. Hydralazine 25–50 mg bd PO or 5–10 mg IV over 10 minutes. Hydralazine is rarely used as monotherapy, but it can be added to some of the other agents. It is still a useful drug for the treatment of hypertensive crises in pregnancy.

Diuretics: generally diuretics should be avoided in pregnancy, if possible, because pregnant women are already oliguric and further intravascular volume depletion might impair uteroplacental perfusion. Diuretics can be used judiciously in small doses, particularly in salt-sensitive hypertensive women.

Calcium channel blockers (CCB): It is almost never appropriate to use the sublingual form of nifedipine. This class of antihypertensive drugs may be used during pregnancy, avoid at labour. CCB are widely used in patients with established renal disease, particularly in those with kidney transplants on calcineurin inhibitors.

Adverse effects of ACE inhibitors: Advise pregnant women to stop the ACE inhibitor if they are attempting pregnancy or as soon as they miss their period. These classes of drugs should not be used in pregnancy, especially in the early pregnancy as they may interfere with fetal kidney development.

Pregnancy in women with polyarteritis nodosa or scleroderma with renal involvement appears to be disastrous due to associated hypertension, which frequently becomes malignant. Prognosis is poor for fetus but also for mother, and pregnancy should be terminated at an early stage.

Lupus nephritis in pregnancy

(See Systemic Lupus Erythematosus and Lupus nephritis; Antiphospholipid antibody syndrome)

Maintenance therapy for lupus nephritis and flare of lupus in pregnancy is azathioprine and prednisolone. They are relatively safe medications in pregnancy. Pregnancy may stimulate disease activity in SLE, including nephritis leading to deterioration in renal function. Unlike many autoimmune diseases, this exacerbation can occur at any time during pregnancy, not just in the puerperium. Immunosuppressive treatment doses should be increased if there is clinical and serological evidence of increasing disease activity.

Renal transplant and pregnancy

(See under Transplantation)

Urinary Tract Infection in pregnancy

Asymptomatic bacteriuria: antibiotic therapy of asymptomatic bacteriuria effectively appears to reduce the rate of pyelonephritis and low birth weight. Short course (three days) antibiotic therapy is usually effective in eradicating the symptomatic bacteriuria of pregnancy. The following regimens are recommended: amoxicillin (500 mg tds PO for three days), or augmentin (500 mg bd PO for three days; or nitrofurantoin (50 mg qds PO for 3 – 7 days, but not near term or in nursing mothers). Starting therapy with cephalosporin (cefalexin, 250 mg qds PO for three days) has been recommended recently because a significant number of E. coli infections are resistant to ampicillin.

Women with refractory bacteriuria should have two weeks course of therapy.

Maintenance therapy is recommended for women with persistent bacteriuria (i.e., ≥2 positive urine cultures). Nitrofurantoin (50 to 100 mg orally at bedtime) for the duration of the pregnancy is one option, or cephalexin (250 to 500 mg orally at bedtime) may also be used.

Cystitis: A urine culture in patients with signs and symptoms suggestive of cystitis should be sent to the laboratory and empirical antibiotic therapy started. Empirical treatment regimens include amoxicillin (250 mg tds), nitrofurantoin (50 – 100 mg bd PO), or cephalexin (250 mg qds PO or 500 mg bd); if there is no available urine culture and sensitivity; each of these drugs is given for three to seven days. Other regimens, which have a broader spectrum of activity, include augmentin (500 mg bd or 250 mg tds PO), co-trimoxazole 960 mg bd PO (but not in the third trimester of pregnancy or near the term as it may precipitate kernicterus in the newborn), and cefalexin 250 mg qds or 500 mg tds PO. Administer these drugs for three to seven days.

If urine culture is done, therapy should be adjusted according to the antimicrobial drug sensitivity.

Penicillins, nitrofurantoin and cephalosporins are safe in pregnancy

Nitrofurantoin should be avoided after 36th week of gestation due to potential risk of hemolysis if the fetus is G6PD deficient

Fluoroquinolones should be avoided in pregnancy

Tetracyclines are contraindicated in pregnancy because they deposit in fetal bone and may also cause severe reactions in mother including liver failure

Sulphonamides should not be used near term because they precipitate kernicterus in the newborn. Anti folic acid activity of trimethoprim has been associated with cleft palate (in animals) and this drug should also be avoided at least before midpregnancy

Pyelonephritis: pyuria is present in virtually all women with this disorder. Blood cultures are positive in 10 to 20 percent of patients. Pyelonephritis in pregnant women has traditionally been treated with hospitalization and intravenous antibiotics until the woman is afebrile for 24 to 48 hours and symptomatically improved. One of the regiment is: IV cefazolin (0.5 – 1 g bd IM/IV) followed at discharge by cephalexin (250 mg qds PO or 500 mg bd - tds PO for 10 days). An outpatient regimen consisting of ceftriaxone 1 g daily IM for two days followed by oral cephalexin (250 mg qds or 500 mg bd for 10 days) has comparable effects.

Inpatient treatment: parenteral beta lactams or gentamicin are the preferred antibiotics (adjust doses if there is renal impairment). Some of the regimens for treatment of acute pyelonephritis in pregnancy include: Ceftriaxone 1 g od IM; gentamicin 3–5 mg/kg od; or gentamicin 1 mg/kg tds; ampicillin 1–2 g four times/day. Symptoms that persist for more than 48 hours, despite adequate intravenous antibiotic therapy, require further evaluation with a renal ultrasound to assess for perinephric abscess, renal calculi and/or obstruction to drainage (pyonephrosis).

Intravenous treatment should continue until the patient is afebrile for 48 hours. Inpatient therapy is followed by an outpatient course of appropriate antibiotics to complete 10 to 14 days of treatment. Low dose antimicrobial prophylaxis, such as nitrofurantoin (50 to 100 mg at night PO) or cephalexin (125 mg at night PO), and periodic urinary surveillance for infection are recommended for the remainder of the pregnancy to prevent recurrence.

Thrombotic thrombocytopenic purpura and Haemolytic-uraemic syndrome

These conditions may develop post-partum and be associated with renal failure. Treatment is the same as in described under HUS and TTP.

RETROPERITONEAL FIBROSIS

There are a number of surgical treatments including ureterolysis, transposition of ureters laterally, omental wrapping of ureters, intraperitoneal placement of ureters etc. Trend is to place ureteric stents.

Primary treatment is surgical: restore renal function and relieve obstruction either with percutaneous nephrostomy tubes or indwelling double-J catheters (stent) situated in the renal pelves and bladder. This nonoperative approach may stabilize the critically ill patient with renal failure prior to definitive surgical exploration or medical therapy. Ureteric stents should be replaced periodically. If retroperitoneal fibrosis is due to aortic aneurysm, deal with it!

Medical therapies include steroids eg pulse Methylprednisolone 1 g IV od for three consecutive days followed by oral steroids (Prednisolone 60 mg od PO and taper to 20 mg od PO). There is a high incidence of recurrence once steroids stopped.

Steroids can be combined with immunosuppressive agents such as azathioprine 100 – 150 mg od PO or mycophenolate mofetil.

Possibly offending drugs should be discontinued (practolol, methysergide).

RENAL ARTERY STENOSIS (RAS)

(Ischaemic Renal Disease, Ischaemic nephropathy, Renovascular Hypertension)

Revascularization may be indicated if the degree of stenosis is higher than 80–85%. In patients with normal renal function this procedure may prevent renal insufficiency. When renal insufficiency is present and the objective is recovery of renal function with prevention of further deterioration in renal function, the prognosis is better if there is serum creatinine < 350 micmol/l, renal length > 9 cm and a renal biopsy showing well-preserved glomeruli with minimal interstitial scarring.

Revascularization may be achieved by surgical renal revascularization or percutaneous transluminal renal artery angioplasty (PTRA), the latter with or without renal artery stenting.

If the goal of intervention in renal artery disease is primarily to improve BP control, interventional strategy for atherosclerotic lesions that involve the ostium, surgery is the preferred treatment. Stents for the treatment of ostial renal artery stenosis are now being employed with improved technical success. If renal artery disease and presumed renovascular hypertension are due to one of fibrous dysplasias, in particular medial fibroplasias, PTRA is usually the interventional modality of choice.

Control of hypertension preferably with ACEI or AIIRA; significant rise in serum creatinine or hyperkalaemia may limit their utility. In this case calcium channel blockers are the most useful and best tolerated agents.

Strict control of serum lipids with statins.

The more common problem of renal failure may be due to cholesterol microemboli (See CHOLESTEROL CRYSTAL ATHEROEMBOLIC RENAL DISEASE)

RHABDOMYOLYSIS

Start therapy as early as possible with the aim of preventing ARF. Monitor BP, CVP and urine output!

Start early massive intravascular volume repletion to compensate for third volume spacing of fluid in the injured muscle: isotonic saline infusions at 1 – 1.5L/h; Mannitol 10 g could be added once hypovolaemia corrected, if the patient is not anuric. Maximum amount of mannitol should not exceed 200 g/d. Continue saline infusion until blood pressure is stable. Once urine flow is established (to 200–300 mL/hour) change to one-half isotonic saline or D5% to which 40 mEq sodium bicarbonate (total 200 – 300 mEq for the first day). Be careful not to precipitate pulmonary oedema with over vigorous rehydration.

Alkalinisation, infusion of mannitol, and urine output >300 ml/h should be continued until urine is free of myoglobin. Alkalinisation of urine with sodium bicarbonate infusion may reduce the risk of tubular obstruction with myoglobin casts.

Monitor carefully serum sodium and calcium concentration. Hypocalcaemia may be severe during the acute phase; rebound hypercalcaemia is common during the recovery phase and resolves spontaneously.

Surgical opinion for compartmental syndrome should be sought urgently. Sustained intracompartmental pressures indicate the need for fasciotomy to prevent irreversible peripheral nerve injury by muscle swelling in tight fascial planes.

When renal failure ensues despite mentioned measures, dialysis will be required for control of hyperkalaemia and hyperphosphataemia. Dialysis modality may be slow VVHDF or daily haemodialysis. The patients usually recover renal function after a period of dialysis.

SEPSIS AND SEPTIC SHOCK

Sepsis associated with ARF has high mortality of >70%. The cornerstones of treatment in this condition are fluids and vasopressors, as well as antibiotics and other treatments aimed at the underlying sepsis.

Intravenous volume expanders, packed red blood cells and vasoactive agents are often required for correction of hypotension.

Fluid therapy should be administered in rapidly infused boluses (one to two litres in the first one hour). Intravenous fluid challenges can be repeated until blood pressure, tissue perfusion, and oxygen delivery are optimised. Clinical trials have not demonstrated a clear-cut superiority of colloid over crystalloid in the treatment of septic shock. Therefore saline solutions are generally preferred in patients with severe hypovolemia not due to bleeding. It is not possible to precisely predict the total fluid deficit in a given patient with hypovolaemic shock, particularly if fluid loss continues due to bleeding or third space sequestration. It may be necessary to give >20 mL/kg rapidly initially in an attempt to rapidly restore tissue perfusion. Further fluids should optimally be given while monitoring the central venous pressure (goal 8 – 12 mm Hg) or pulmonary capillary wedge pressure. In mechanically ventilated patients a higher central venous pressure of 12 – 15 mm Hg is recommended to account for the increased intrathoracic pressure. Fluid repletion should continue at the initial rapid rate as long as the cardiac filling pressures and the systemic blood pressure remain low. Saline solutions are generally preferred in patients with severe volume depletion not due to bleeding: they seem to be as safe and as effective as colloid-containing solutions.

If during the first 6 hours of resuscitation central venous pressure of 8 – 12 mm Hg or mixed venous oxygen saturation of 70% is not achieved, then transfuse packed red blood cells to achieve a hematocrit >30%. Blood transfusion is indicated if Hgb <7 g/L, if the patient has active bleeding or myocardial ischemia. Aim to get Hgb 10 – 12 g/dL.

Vasopressors are indicated as second line agents in the treatment of severe sepsis and septic shock in patients who are hypotensive despite adequate fluid replacement or who develop pulmonary oedema. A variety of agents with different peripheral and cardiac actions are available. Either noradrenaline (norepinephrine) or dopamine through central catheter is the first-choice vasopressor agent to correct hypotension in septic shock. Noradrenaline is more potent than dopamine. The doses of some are as follows:

Noradrenaline dose 0.5 – 5 μg/min is preferable to dopamine.

Dopamine dose 1–20 μg/kg/min ("renal dose" 2 – 5 μg/kg/min; vasopressor dose up to 20 μg/kg/min). The available data do not support administration of low doses of dopamine to maintain or improve renal function.

Adrenaline dose 0.5 – 10 μg/min is an alternative to noradrenaline.

Phenylnephrine dose 10–500 μg/kg/min is a pure alpha-adrenergic agonist may be particularly useful when tachycardia or arrhythmias preclude the use of agents with beta-adrenergic activity.

Vasopressin use may be considered in patients with refractory shock despite adequate fluid resuscitation and high dose conventional vasopressors. It should be administered at infusion rates of 0.01 – 0.04 units.min.

Dobutamine is the first-choice inotrope for patients with low cardiac output in the presence of adequate fluid resuscitation. The dose of dobutamine: 2.5 – 10 μg/kg/min; it can cause a modest vasodilatation therefore should not be administered as a single agent in patients with septic shock

Inspired oxygen >35% should be supplied to all patients with sepsis to maintain oxygen saturation >90%. Oxygenation should be monitored using continuous pulse oximetry.

High-dose loop diuretics should be used cautiously in critically ill patients with ARF. Intravascular volume depletion should be corrected before and during administration of diuretics to reduce the risk of further decrease in kidney perfusion pressure.

Continuous bicarbonate infusion is indicated in patients with acidosis (blood pH 7.2).

Start IV antibiotic therapy as soon as appropriate cultures have been collected (adjust doses for renal impairment). An empirical regimen of broad-spectrum antimicrobial agents should be instituted as early as possible; antibiotics should be adjusted as culture results become available. Potential gram-negative pathogens are generally covered with two effective agents from different antibiotic classes, usually beta-lactam (Meropenem 1 g IV every 8 h as a 5 min bolus) + aminoglycoside gentamicin 3 mg/kg/d IV (check blood level, trough level should be <2 mg/L). Aminoglycoside could be substituted with Ciprofloxacin 200 – 400 mg bd IV or PO.

The other option is a third generation cephalosporin such as Ceftriaxone 1 g od IV, Cefotaxime 2x1 g IV, ceftazidime 1–2 g bd IV or Cefuroxime 1.5 g tds IV.

Antibiotics such as: carbapenem, ceftriaxone, cefipime, aminoglycosides do not have the propensity to provoke septic shock due to release of bacterial endotoxins.

The duration of antibiotic therapy should typically be 7 – 10 days and guided by clinical response.

Dialytic treatment, if needed, may be either continuous renal replacement therapy or intermittent (daily or alternate days) hemodialysis.

Recombinant protein C has been recently recently approved for treatment of severe septic shock. This treatment should be applied early, within first 48 hours of sepsis, it can cause bleeding and should not be given if platelet count <30×10^9/L.

Following initial stabilization of patients with severe sepsis, monitor serum glucose concentration, maintain blood glucose <150 mg/dL

(8.3 mmol/L) and give continuous infusion of insulin when necessary.

Steroid therapy in septic shock is controversial, but small dose of hydrocortisone (50 mg qds slow IV infusion) may improve survival in patients with relative adrenal insufficiency or patients with septic shock who, despite adequate fluid replacement, require vasopressor therapy to maintain adequate blood pressure.

In patients with severe sepsis, platelets should be administered when counts are <5,000/mm^3 (5 x 10^9/L) regardless of apparent bleeding. Platelet transfusion may be considered when counts are 5,000 – 30,000 mm^3 (5 – 30 x 10^9/L) and there is significant risk of bleeding.

Severe sepsis patients should receive deep vein thrombosis prophylaxis with either low-dose unfractionated heparin or low molecular weight heparin. For patients who have a contraindication for heparin use, the use of mechanical DVT prophylaxis device is indicated.

Strees ulcer prophylaxis with H2-receptor antagonist should be given to all patients with severe sepsis: Ranitidine initial slow IV injection of 50 mg, then continuous infusion 125 – 250 micrograms/kg/hour. When oral feeding commences ranitidine could be given orally in thedose of 150 mg bd PO.

SYSTEMIC LUPUS ERYTHEMATOSUS (Lupus nephritis)

In patients with mild forms of Lupus nephritis treatment is usually directed at extrarenal manifestations of SLE. Moderate doses of corticosteroids are administered, with possible addition of azathioprine if initial response is poor.

Current therapy of severe proliferative Lupus nephritis (according to clinical manifestations, laboratory parameters and histology) includes cytotoxic agents plus corticosteroids. It is conventional to divide the treatment into induction and maintenance phases. The following regiment is based on the trials at the National Institutes of Health:

Induction phase: cyclophosphamide once/month for 6 months in the dose of $0.75 g/m^2$ BSA (0.5 to 1.0 g per square meter of body surface area) if creatinine clearance >40 ml/min (the Mosteller formula for Body Surface Area is recommended and the most frequently used by the body surface area calculator). If nadir WBC >4000 increase next dose of cyclophosphamide by 0.25 g. If Cr.Cl. <40 ml/min, reduce cyclophosphamide to 0.5 g/m² BSA. Titrate the dose of cyclophosphamide to maintain a leucocyte count of no less than 2000 cells per cubic milliliter.

Cyclophosphamide should be dissolved in 150 ml isotonic saline and infused IV over 60 min.

Consider sperm and egg storage in sperm/egg bank and counsel patients about likelihood of infertility/sterility after this treatment. There is some evidence that timing of pulses of cyclophosphamide in female patients to coincide with menstrual period may reduce the risk of subsequent infertility.

After an intravenous dose of cyclophosphamide the toxic urinary metabolites fall to non-toxic levels within 8–12 hours. Therefore urine output should be maintained (where possible, subject to renal function) at 100 mls/hour.

At the time of cyclophosphamide infusion:
- Induce diuresis with copious oral fluids or IV administration of 5% dextrose and 0.45% isotonic saline 250 ml/hr for 10 hours, and then reduce to 150 ml/hour for another 8 hours.
- To prevent haemorrhagic cystitis give MESNA 20% of the total cyclophosphamide dose, every 3 hours, orally
- To prevent nausea and vomiting give Ondansetron 4–8 mg 4 hours before cyclophosphamide and further doses 8 and 12 hours after cyclophosphamide infusion. Metoclopramide 10 mg IM could also prevent nausea and vomiting.

Prednisolone is given in conjunction with cyclophosphamide at 0.5–1 mg/kg/day, not more than 60 mg/day, for 4–6 weeks. After 4–6 weeks gradually reduce by 5 mg every 2 weeks until reached 20 mg, then reduce by 2.5 mg every 4 weeks to maintenance dose of 10 mg/day.

In very severe forms of lupus nephritis combination therapy of monthly pulses methylprednisolone (500–1000 mg IV) plus monthly pulses of cyclophosphamide IV accompanied by a low dose oral prednisolone for six months, then quarterly resulted in even higher remission rate, but was accompanied with a higher incidence of side-effects.

One of the newer regimens with comparable efficacy to high dose pulse cyclophosphamide is a short course, low dose cyclophosphamide as an alternative remission-inducing treatment for proliferative Lupus nephritis without the need for IV antiemetics and forced hydration: 500 mg cyclophosphamide pulse as 30 min IV infusion fortnightly, in total six pulses (3 g total dose). This protocol includes one pulse dose of methyprednisolone at the start and low dose oral prednisolone during the whole course of treatment.

<u>Maintenance phase</u>: after six monthly pulses, one infusion of "pulse" dose of cyclophosphamide give quarterly i.e. every 3 months to the end of second year (6 further pulses) or 1 year after remission was achieved.

Following therapy with IV cyclophsophamide, give remission maintenance therapy with either oral azathioprine (1 to 3 mg/kg/d) or mycophenolate mofetil (250 mg bd and increase to 1 g bd) for one to three years.

Other therapeutic options, for less severe forms of Lupus nephritis or for patients who could not tolerate or are refractory to steroids, cyclophosphamide or azathioprine therapy includes:

- Cyclosporine in the doses of 4 – 6 mg/kg/day. These currently used doses of cyclosporine are accompanied by less nephrotoxicity or other side-effects than previously used high doses of >8 mg/kg/day. Cyclosporine monotherapy is much less effective then combination of cyclosporine and other immunosuppressives.
- Mycophenolate mofetil 250 mg bd and increase to 1 g bd + low dose of steroids.
- IV immunoglobulin gamma (0.4 g/kg/d for 5 days) on a monthly basis could ameliorate LN with improvement of proteinuria, creatinine clearance, serologic markers of disease activity and renal histology

Patients with membranous lupus nephritis with deteriorating renal functions and massive edema should be treated as proliferative lupus nephritis (steroids plus cyclophosphamide) or steroids plus cyclosporine. Limited experience to date with cyclosporine in patients with membranous Lupus nephritis suggests that most patients will experience reduction in proteinuria.

For milder lupus nephritis use low dose of steroids and azathioprine 2.5 mg/kg/day.

Hydroxychloroquine 200–400 mg/day is good for extra-renal lupus (lupus arthritis, skin lupus etc).

Use ACEI for control of proteinuria and statins for hyperlipidaemia.

Plasmapheresis can be used in selected patients with severe proliferative LN, patients with anticardiolipin antibodies and thrombotic thrombocytopenic purpura. Plasmpheresis should be synchronized with cytotoxic drugs.

Maintenance therapy: there are no strict guidelines for maintenance therapy after remission was induced. Common practice is to give the maintenance therapy for 12–18 months at least.

Newer therapies of SLE

Newer therapies that are still in process of development, some are still at the stage of animal experiments and will not be described in more detail. These treatments might be good for the patient refractory to "classic" therapies, patient with frequent flares of SLE, patient with serious side-effects of intolerance to "classic"therapies. We would like just to mention some of them. They are:

- LJP 394 100 mg IV once a week (reduces flares of SLE in patients with high affinity anti-DNA antibodies)
- anti -CD40 ligand
- rituximab (monoclonal antibody against B-cell specific antigen CD20) 375 mg/M^2 IV weekly for 4 weeks combined with cyclophosphamide IV monthly and steroids
- blockers of interferon-gamma
- IL-10
- anti-C5 antibody
- immunoablative therapy

Pregnancy and SLE

Exacerbations of lupus nephritis are common during and after pregnancy. Care of the pregnant LN patient should be shared between obstetrician and nephrologist.

Women with lupus nephritis should be encouraged to delay pregnancy until the disease can be rendered inactive for at least six months. Mothers should be assessed for disease activity at least once each trimester, and more often if SLE is active.

Women who show evidence of increased serological activity but remain asymptomatic should be monitored more closely. Do not initiate therapy for serological findings alone.

Corticosteroids are relatively safe to use during pregnancy. Prednisolone crosses the placenta at very low concentration whereas dexamethasone and betamethasone reach the fetus at higher concentration.

Low doses (less than 10 mg/day) of prednisolone may be sufficient to control the disease activity.

Azathioprine may be used cautiously.

Patients with a significant flare of lupus nephritis should be treated with high-dose prednisolone; plus antihypertensive medication if necessary (hydralazine, methyldopa and calcium channel blockers (See hypertension and pregnancy).

Angiotensin converting enzyme inhibitors and some beta-blockers are contraindicated in pregnancy.

Cyclophosphamide and methotrexate are contraindicated during pregnancy.

Hydroxychloroquine should be avoided in pregnancy and breastfeeding.

NSAIDs are safe in first and second trimester but should be discontinued in the last trimester of pregnancy.

Thrombocytopaenia during lupus pregnancies may have multiple causes, including antiplatelet antibodies, toxaemia, and antiphospholipid antibodies. Treatment includes high dose prednisolone.

Although the presence of antiphospholipid antibodies does not necessarily predict fetal loss, patients with SLE and antiphospholipid antibodies appear to be at increased risk for spontaneous miscarriage. Fetal loss typically occurs in the second trimester. For treatment see Antiphospholipid antibody syndrome and pregnancy.

If the fetus develops incomplete or complete heart block, prenatal treatment should be considered with the administration of steroids that cross placenta beginning at week 23, and persisting through the end of pregnancy.

Following delivery, the neonatologist should be prepared to insert a cardiac pacemaker in infants, especially so if the heart rate before delivery is less than 50 per minute.

THROMBOTIC THROMBOCYTOPAENIC PURPURA AND HAEMOLYTIC URAEMIC SYNDROME (TTP and HUS)

Plasma exchange or plasma infusion should always be tried in TTP and may also be useful in adult HUS (if only by allowing infusion of large volumes of fresh frozen plasma, FFP). These procedures are seldom effective in secondary forms of TTP and HUS where specific therapy should be started as soon as diagnosis is established.

The infusion of FFP: equivalent to one plasma volume (30 mL/kg body weight) over the first 24 h and about 20 mL/kg/d thereafter.
Plasma exchange: replace one to two plasma volumes up to 4 L/session/d.
Replacement fluid fresh frozen plasma or cryosupernatant.
Give diuretic or perform ultrafiltration to avoid fluid overload.
In addition to plasma exchange steroids (Prednisolone 60 mg/d PO) are possibly effective in treatment of TTP. Prednisolone should be tapered by 5 mg/week.
Treatment should be continued until complete remission is achieved (platelet count > 100×10^9/l, LDH normal).

TRANSPLANTATION (RENAL)

Acute rejection

After diagnosing acute graft rejection (clinical and laboratory data plus graft biopsy) for the first episode of rejection (cellular rejection) give methylprednisolone 500–1000 mg IV over 30–60 minutes, daily for three to five days. This should be diluted in 50 mL of either 0.9% saline or 5% glucose. The dose of methylprednisolone depends on the intensity of rejection and body weight of the patient (500 mg if patient <50 kg; 1 g if patient >50 kg). Improvement is usually rapid. After completing these 3–5 days of pulse methylprednisolone, the maintenance dose of corticosteroid is resumed at the prerejection level or is increased to 20 mg/day for 4–6 weeks and then tapered to baseline level over a few days. Prophylactic antacid /H2 blockers and oral antifungal therapy are generally recommended.

In follow-up, now that several alternative anti-rejection agents are available, many centres change the maintenance regimen on the grounds that the existing regimen has failed to prevent rejection. First, ensure compliance and check that adequate therapeutic blood levels have been achieved previously. If not, an option is to change the dose of cyclosporin. If rejection has occurred despite adequate blood levels of cyclosporin, many centres would change to tacrolimus. If azathioprine has been used to maximal dose of 2.5 mg/kg/day, consider a change to mycophenolate mofetil.

In steroid resistant cases, i.e. if serum creatinine remains elevated for more than 20% above baseline after 7 days, proceed to antibody therapy.

Antibody therapy for acute graft rejection

Monoclonal antibody therapy: OKT3 5 mg daily as IV bolus for 10–14 days. Patient should be euvolaemic, ensure this by diuretics or ultrafiltration if the patient is volume-overloaded. Give pre-medication (30 minutes before infusion of antibody) before first and second dose consisting of 100 mg hydrocortisone, chlorphenamine maleate 10 mg IV/IM (Piriton) and paracetamol 500 mg PO. Monitor vital signs every 15 minutes for 2 hours, then every 30 minutes for another 2 hours. Premedication is not necessary for the remainder of the course, use only paracetamol PRN for fever.

Monitor T-cell subsets, target <$50/mm^3$. During the course of antibody therapy reduce prednisolone to 0.1 mg/kg/day, reduce azathioprine to 25–50 mg/day, and reduce the dose of mycophenolate mofetil. CsA therapy is usually discontinued at the start of OKT3 treatment and restarted 3 days before termination of OKT3. Re-start prednisolone with scheduled dose after second dose of antibody.

Polyclonal antibody therapy is used either for prophylaxis (induction therapy) or primary and secondary therapy of acute rejection. Polyclonal therapy is also used to reverse rebound rejection following OKT3 administration in patients with high titers of anti-mouse antibodies which limit retreatment with OKT3.

Anti-thymocyte gamma globulin (horse polyclonal globulin) use 10–15 mg/kg daily in 500 mL 5% dextrose or normal saline as IV infusion over 4–8 hours, or Thymoglobulin (Rabbit) 1–1.5 mg/kg/day. Duration of therapy 7–14 days. Dilute antibody in 500 mL 5% dextrose/normal saline and infuse over 4–8 hours in peripheral vein. Adding Solu-Cortef 20 mg and heparin 1,000 u to the infusion may prevent vein thrombosis. Premedication (methylprednisolone 30 mg IV, diphenhydramine hydrochloride 50 mg IV and paracetamol 500 mg orally) should be given 30 min before the infusion.

Monitor vital signs every 15 minutes for 2 hours, then every 30 minutes for another 2 hours. Azathioprine and mycophenolate should be discontinued during the course of antibody infusions, cyclosporine or tacrolimus should be omitted during the course and oral prednisolone is replaced by methylprednisolone in the premedication.

Anticoagulation

Before surgery:

Prescribe Enoxaparin (Clexane 20 mg (2000 units) SC od with premedication.

If patient was therapeutically anticoagulated with warfarin, this should be reversed:
- If INR >1.5 two units of FFP (600 mL) IV over 1 hour + Vit K 1 mg IV stat (if INR 1.5–3), or Vit K 2 mg IV stat (if INR >3).

After surgery:

Check INR, if INR <2 prescribe Enoxaparin (Clexane) 40 mg SC od. Do not re-introduce warfarin in the first week after transplantation if the transplant is not functioning, since biopsy will be required.
When clinically appropriate (usually after day 7, re-introduce normal dose of warfarin. Do not re-load with warfarin. Continue Enoxaparin until INR <2.

Antimicrobial prophylaxis

Antimicrobial prophylaxis can be administered for various reasons:

1. at the time of renal transplant operation, prior to skin incision: prescribe Cefazolin 1 g IV or Flucloxacillin 1 g IV at induction and 6 hours later (omit if allergic)

2. perioperative surgical antibiotic prophylaxis with one of broad spectrum antibiotic to reduce the risk of wound infection with antibiotics directed against skin pathogens and urinary tract infection pathogens:
   - Augmentin 1.2 g IV single dose (for colorectal surgery, cholecystectomy etc)
   - Piperacillin 2 g IV single dose
   - Tazocin 2.25–4.5 g IV two doses 8 hours apart
   - Imipenem, Meropenem 500 mg IV over 5 minutes every 12 hours
   - Vancomycin 1 g slow IV over 100 min plus Cephalexin 250 mg qds PO or 500 mg bd PO or
   - 1st generation cephalosporins (Cefazolin 1.0 g bd IM or IV) or
   - beta-lactams
   - single dose of aminoglycoside 5 mg/kg (in genitor-urinary surgery)
   - Teicoplanin 400 mg IV bd for 3 doses, then 200 mg od (high risk patients such as patients with prosthetic valves).

Antibiotics should be administered perioperatively and discontinued after 2–3 days after operation to minimize the risk of resistant microorganism growth.

3. co-trimoxazole for prevention of Pneumocystis carinii pneumonia, urinary tract infections, sepsis (See UTI in Transplant – renal)

4. CMV prophylaxis to prevent infection of CMV negative recipients of CMV positive donor (See Cytomegalovirus infection).

Immunosuppressed patients on high doses of antibiotics or prolonged courses of antibiotic therapy should have antifungal prophylaxis (Nystatin, Fluconazole, Amphotericin B lozenge etc)

Bone disease

Most of the bone loss occurs during the first 6 months after transplant. High-risk patients are menopausal women, anyone with previous fractures or known osteoporosis, patients with hyperparathyroidism before transplantation, diabetics etc. Patients with significant bone loss on DEXA scan are candidates for treatment with oral calcium and vitamin D supplementation. If there are no signs (bone biopsy, biochemical markers etc) of adynamic bone disease, then biphosphonates are indicated.

A number of biphosphonates are available:
Alendronate 5 mg od PO or Fosamax 70 mg Once Weekly PO
Pamidronate 0.5 mg/kg in 500 ml 0.9% saline IV two doses one month apart.

Cervical smears in female renal transplant recipients

Immunocompromised patients are at increased risk of cervical carcinoma. We recommend cervical smears (and any necessary follow-up treatment) before going onto the transplant list and at annual intervals after transplantation

Chronic allograft nephropathy

There is no definite treatment for biopsy proven chronic allograft nephropathy. However, there is some evidence that discontinuation or reduced dose (to 50%) of calcineurin inhibitors (cyclosporine or tacrolimus) may slow the rate of loss of renal function in patients with deteriorating renal function due to chronic allograft nephropathy. Immunosuppression support should be maintained by substituting for azathioprine, or adding or continuing and/or increasing the dose of mycophenolate mofetil to 0.5 – 1 g bd. Low-dose steroids ≈ 0.1 mg/kg/d prednisolone should be given.

The strategy described should be considered as part of other therapeutic modalities including intensive control of blood pressure (See Hypertension), glycemia and cholesterol metabolism.

Conversion of cyclosporine to tacrolimus has no proven beneficial effect in patients with chronic allograft nephropathy.

Cytomegalovirus infection

Stop azathioprine or mycophenolate mofetil if there is leucopenia. Restart azathioprine when WBC over $4{,}000\text{--}5{,}000 \times 10^9/l$.
Therapeutic treatment of established CMV disease is primarily with the antiviral agent Ganciclovir. Ganciclovir 5 mg/kg twice daily IV for 3 weeks, dependent on blood viral load (DNA), then reduce to 5

mg/kg once daily IV until disappearance of viral RNA in PCR, then 750–1000 mg two to three times per day PO for two to 12 weeks.

The dose of Ganciclovir can be adjusted according to creatinine clearance:

Creatinine clearance 50 – 75 ml/min, Ganciclovir 2.5 mg bd IV
Creatinine clearance 25–50 ml/min: Ganciclovir 2.5 mg od IV
Creatinine clearance <25 mL/min, Ganciclovir 1.25 mg/kg od IV

For treatment of severe CMV infection (sepsis, pneumonia, gastrointestinal involvement) the addition of hyperimmune CMV Ig (100 mg/kg IV every other day for five days) may be beneficial. For full control of the disease the duration of therapy is 100 days.

Valganciclovir has oral bioavailability of nearly 70% (compared with 7% for oral ganciclovir) and at doses of 450 to 900 mg produces ganciclovir levels that are similar to intravenous administration of ganciclovir at 2.5 to 5 mg/kg. Adult dosing of valganciclovir in induction phase 900 mg bd PO for 21 days. The dose of valganciclovir should be reduced in renal impairment. Following induction treatment continue with maintenance therapy 900 mg od PO for up to 100 days post-transplantation.

Foscarnet may also be used but is nephrotoxic and inconvenient to administer. It is used primarily when ganciclovir resistance is detected.

Prevention of CMV disease:
- Oral Ganciclovir is highly effective for prevention in the dose 1000 mg three times daily for 12 weeks starting posttransplant.
- Valaciclovir (2 g four times daily) is replacing Ganciclovir in prevention of CMV infection among high-risk renal transplant patients.
- Valganciclovir 900 mg od PO is at least as effective as oral ganciclovir thrice daily for preventing CMV disease in high risk (donor CMV+/recipient CMV-) transplant recipients.

Delayed graft function

Ensure patency of urethral catheter (flush gently with 50 mL of 0.9% saline to exclude blockage).

Check renal scans for graft perfusion, ultrasound of the graft for obstruction, urine leak, Doppler ultrasound for renal vasculature and patency.

If patient is hypervolaemic (oedema, high CVP, pulmonary congestion on chest X-rays) give up to 200 mg Frusemide IV.

If the patient is hypovolaemic saline should be given in boluses of 250 to 500 ml.

Indications for haemodialysis in transplant recipient are the same as in any patient with postoperative renal dysfunction. Avoid hypotension as it may perpetuate graft dysfunction. A no-heparin protocol should be used. Ultrafiltration should be avoided to prevent hypotension. A 2 – 3 hour haemodialysis is usually adequate.

If hyperkalemia is treated conservatively (calcium gluconate IV, glucose + insulin IV) calcium resonium or resonium A should not be used in early postoperative period because of risk of colonic dilatation and perforation.

Cut the dose of calcineurin inhibitor, i.e reduce the dose to half (tacrolimus to 0.05 mg/kg PO bd or ciclosporin to 0.2 mg/kg PO bd). Instead of azathioprine use mycophenolate mofetil 1 g PO bd if given concomitantly with ciclosporin or 0.5 g PO bd if given concomitantly with tacrolimus. Increase dose of prednisolone to 40 mg/day.

When transplanted kidney has started to function as indicated by symptomatic fall in serum creatinine increase the dose of tacrolimus to the standard 0.1 mg/kg PO bd or cyclosporine to 4 mg/kg PO bd respectively. Continue mycophenolate mofetil for 3 months before switching to azathioprine. Reduce prednisolone to standard dose.

Diabetes mellitus (post transplant)

Life-style changes (diet) and exercise.

Oral antidiabetic drugs if blood glucose <250 mg/dl:
- sulphonylureas (Gliclazide, Glipizide)
- biguanides (Metformin) could be used with caution as for other patients without renal transplant.
- thiazolidinediones (pioglitazone and others): either alone (if patient is unable to take metformin or sulphonylurea), or in combination with sulphonylurea or insulin, or with metformin. Edema without proteinuria is a side-effect that we noticed in some patients on rosiglitazone.

Treatment with insulin (Insulin glargine or HumalogMix 25) is needed if blood glucose >250 mg/dl and if all the efforts to modify lifestyle and the use of oral hypoglycemic agents have failed.

Diuretics (intraoperatively)

Intraoperative diuretics are given shortly before revascularization of kidney graft: Frusemide 250 mg IV and Mannitol 20% 100 mL IV.

Fluids

It is important to optimize renal perfusion immediately after transplantation. CVP line should be inserted and CVP kept in 8–10 cm range. Prescribe colloid (Gelofusine 500 ml IV PRN) to keep CVP 8–10 cm. Transfuse blood if operative blood loss or blood loss from drains are excessive.

The regime for crystalloid infusion depend on urine output; prescribe 0.45% saline with glucose at a rate equal to previous fluid output + 25 mL (if a patient is hyperglycaemic substitute 0.45% with 0.9% saline).

If urine output is > 200 mL/hour, stop colloid infusion. Reduce crystalloid input to equal total fluid output. Include potassium with replacement crystalloid (40 mmol/L). Check serum potassium at least twice daily and adjust replacement as required.

If urine output stops, flush urinary catheter gently with 50 mL saline to exclude blockage.

Gingival hyperplasia

This common in transplant recipients, exacerbated by poor oral hygiene, cyclosporin and CCB especially nifedipine. Oral hygiene should be optimised prior to transplantation. If gingival hyperplasia is developing CCB should be stopped. If it continues to be troublesome, changing cyclosporin to tacrolimus should be considered.

Case reports suggest that the gingival hyperplasia can be effectively treated with a two-week course of metronidazole (750 mg tds) while cyclosporine is continued.

Azithromycin 500 mg od on day one followed by 250 mg od for three consecutive days. Reduce the dose of cyclosporin as

Azithromycin, like Erythromycin, increases cyclosporine plasma concentration.

The substitution of cyclosporine with tacrolimus or Sirolimus was found to significantly ameliorate gingival hyperplasia without increasing the risk of renal allograft dysfunction or rejection.

Gout/hyperuricemia

Reduction of serum uric acid may be achieved using drug that reduce endogenous production of uric acid through inhibiting xanthine-oxidase activity (allopurinol) or using uricosuric drugs to enhance renal excretion of uric acid.

Allopurinol is one of the antihyperuricemic agents. The starting dose of allopurinol should be reduced in renal insufficiency, usually to 100 mg od. If the patient is on azathioprine, the dose of azathioprine should be lowered to 25 – 50% of the usual dose. Allopurinol increases the blood level and toxicity of azathioprine, but not of mycophenolate mofetil. Therefore, consider replacing azathioprine with mycophenolate mofetil.

Colchicine is effective in the treatment of acute episodes of gout; long-term use may cause gastrointestinal side effects and bone marrow toxicity. The dose of colchicine is 0.5 mg bd initially, followed by 0.5 mg od PO every 2–3 hours until relief of pain is obtained but not for more then 10 days. Stop colchicine if myoneuropathy, diarrhea or vomiting occurs.

Nonsteroidal anti-inflammatory drugs are an effective alternative to colchicine in treating acute attacks or gouty arthritis. However, they should be used extremely cautiously in renal transplant patients. The new cyclooxygenase-2 inhibitors such as celecoxib (100 mg bd) may be less likely to induce renal side effects than conventional NSAID.

New uricosuric agents efficient in treating hyperuricemia in renal transplant patients on cyclosporine are benzofurans such as benziodarone and benzbromarone. They are not universally available.

Hepatitis in renal transplant recipient

Hepatitis B in transplant recipient: Lamivudine 75–100 mg/day PO for more than 6 months.

Hepatitis C: if the patient does not clear virus spontaneously he/she should be considered for 4 months treatment with interferon (IFN) and ribavirin. There is not much data on pegylated IFN. Ribavirin is not recommended for patients with creatinine clearance <50 mL/min. There is evidence that antiviral therapy with interferon may exacerbate acute cellular graft rejection; therefore, graft function should be monitored very closely.

Herpes simplex

Acyclovir 200–400 mg orally five times/day for 10 days; if unable to take PO use 5 mg/kg tds IV usually for 5 days.
Other therapeutic option is Valaciclovir 500 mg bd PO.
(adjust doses for impaired renal function)

Hyperlipidaemia

Hyperlipidaemia is less common in tacrolimus treated patients than in those treated with cyclosporin. Weight reduction if the patient is overweight. Low fat diet.
Statins (atorvastatin 10 – 40 mg od PO) if cholesterol and triglycerides are high
Check CPK (creatine phosphokinase) as rhabdomyolysis was detected in a very small number of patients.
Consider fibrates if the patient is on Sirolimus: Bezafibrate 200 mg tds PO after food
or Gemfibrozil 600 mg bd PO

Hypertension

Life style modification (exercise, cessation of smoking, reduction in body weight), reduced sodium in the diet and all classes of antihypertensive drugs can be used in the treatment of hypertension in renal graft recipients. The following strategies could be used for treatment of hypertension in renal transplant recipient:

- Calcium channel blockers (CCB). Non-dihydropyridine CCB (Diltiazem and Verapamil) increases cyclosporine blood level.
- Low dose thiazide diuretics (if creatinine clearance >25 ml/min) or
- Loop diuretic if GFR low
- Beta-blockers especially in younger patients

- ACEI or angiotensin II receptor antagonist (AIIRA), especially useful if the patient is proteinuric
- Vasodilatators (minoxidil)
- Alpha-blockers (only as a third line of antihypertensive drugs)
- Combination of drugs: diuretic + ACEI or ATIIRA; CCB + beta blocker + diuretic; vasodilatators + beta blocker + diuretic
- Percutaneous transluminal balloon angioplasty if the patient has renal artery stenosis
- Native kidney nephrectomy if uncontrollable hypertension is due to the contribution of native kidneys.

Immunosuppressive medications

The immunosuppressive regimens that we use are tailored to our estimate of the rejection risk of the transplant. For high risk patients (mismatched, highly sensitized) relatively "heavy" immunosuppression is given.

Initial therapy:

Units vary in policy: in the UK the majority of units use "triple therapy" with steroids, azathioprine and calcineurin inhibitor (cyclosporin or tacrolimus) aiming to minimise doses of all three. Other units use "dual therapy" omitting azathioprine.

Azathioprine 1.5–2.5 mg/kg/day PO (round to nearest 25 mg), start the night before operation (at 18.00 hours) and continue afterwards. Azathioprine may be replaced by Mycophenolate mofetil 0.5–1 g PO twice daily (at 06.00 and 18.00 hours)

Steroids: methylprednisolone 250 mg IV is often given at the start of operation and five hours later. After the first postoperative day, continue with oral prednisolone starting with 60 mg od PO on day two; 50 mg od PO on day three; 40 mg od PO on day four; 30 mg od PO on day five. Afterwards reduce the dose of prednisolone depending on patient's renal function. Doses vary, with the trend being to use lower doses than previously (eg 20–30 mg daily PO).

After 4–6 weeks if the patient is rejection-free, reduce dose further to 5–7.5 mg and continue indefinitely (if the patient tolerates or if there are no contraindications or serious side-effects).

Cyclosporin 4–8 mg/kg/single dose immediately before the operation and continue 8–12 mg/kg/day in two divided doses at 06.00 and 18.00 hours. Some centres delay commencement of calcineurin inhibitor until serum creatinine concentration <4 mg/dl (<352 μmol/L). The dose of cyclosporin should be decided according to the blood level twelve hours post dose (trough or C0); recently the manufacturer has advocated C2 monitoring (blood concentration at 2 hours after oral dose) for greater accuracy. Target trough blood levels in the first three weeks 300 ng/ml, in the period up to six months 250 ng/ml, period 6 months – 1 year trough level 200 ng/mL and after one year 150 ng/mL. In maintenance patients C2 concentrations between 500 and 600 ng/mL are well tolerated and provide effective and safe rejection prophylaxis. In the elderly the daily dose of cyclosporin may be lower. If the cyclosporin cannot be given orally, then 1/3 of the total oral daily dose can be given IV. Dilute cyclosporin concentrate (1 mL or 5 mL ampoules of 50 mg/mL) to a concentration of 50 mg in 20–100 mL 5% glucose or normal saline and infuse over 2–6 hours.

When our patients' cyclosporin dose is different in morning and evening we tend to give the bigger dose in the evening and measure the trough level the next day, on the grounds that in longstanding transplants we are more concerned about toxicity than rejection.

Sirolimus can be given with cyclosporin (2 mg od PO to trough level >5 ng/ml) or, if there is a particular reason to avoid calcineurin inhibitor (ciclosporin, tacrolimus). To initiate – Stop ciclosporin/tacrolimus. Next day give sirolimus 8 mg od PO. Then give sirolimus 4 mg od PO. Monitoring – Aim for level of 20–30 ng/mL until month 12, thereafter 15–25 ng/mL.

Tacrolimus is another calcineurin inhibitor and may be a substitute for cyclosporine especially in high/intermediate risk patients. Starting dose of tacrolimus is 0.1 to 0.3 mg/kg/day divided in two doses. Doses should be adjusted to maintain trough blood level (12 hours post-dose) 15–20 ng/ml in the first month, 10–15 ng/ml in the month 1–6, and after that 5–10 ng/ml.

Maintenance therapy (triple therapy) in the period 1 year after transplantation:
1. Prednisolone 0.1 mg/kg/d
2. Cyclosporin to have blood level 100–150 ng/ml

Or
Tacrolimus to have blood level 5–10 ng/ml
Or
Sirolimus 2–5 mg/d or to have blood trough level 10 ng/ml
3. Mycophenolate mofetil 0.5–1.0 g bd PO or to have WBC count > $4000 \times 10^9/l$
Or
Azathioprine 1–2 mg/kg/day or to have WBC count >$5000 \times 10^9/l$

Low dose Ketoconazole 100 mg od PO can be used to reduce calcineurin inhibitor (cyclosporine/tacrolimus) dose (toxicity) and cost in renal transplant recipients.

Induction therapy

Anti-thymocyte globulin (Atgam) and Thymoglobulin could be used also for Induction therapy (Doses see under Acute rejection) or interleukin-2 receptor antagonists:

Basiliximab (Simulect) two IV doses of 20 mg dissolved in 5 mL of water for injection and then made up to 50 mL with 0.9% saline and given as infusion over 30 minutes, the first dose 2 hours preoperatively and the second dose on 4th postoperative day
or
Daclizumab five doses of 1 mg/kg by IV infusion, first dose within 24 hours before operation and subsequent doses every two weeks for a total of 5 doses.

Live donor transplantation protocol
(Cleveland Clinic)

At the start of operation Methylprednisolone 250 mg IV
Five hours later Methylprednisolone 250 mg IV
One-hour later Basiliximab 20 mg
Postoperatively Mycophenolate mofetil 1 g bd

Steroid treatment:
Day 1 post-operation Methylprednisolone 500 mg IV
Day 2 Prednisolone   60/60
Day 2   "   50/50
Day 3   "   40/40
Day 4   "   30/30
Day 5   "   30/15

Day 6	"	30
Day 7 – 14	"	30
Day 15–28	"	25
Day 29–40	"	20
Day 41–54	"	17.5
Day 55–69	"	15
Day 70–84	"	12.5

Afterwards Prednisolone 10–7.5–5 mg depending on the patient's renal function, and other factors that may potentiate steroid side effects.

Start cyclosporin when serum creatinine concentration < 4 mg/dL

Medical fitness for renal transplantation

Policies for assessment of medical fitness of potential renal transplant recipients vary between units and are influenced by resource issues and population characteristics as well as by moral/ethical considerations and the preferences/practices of individual patients, physicians and surgeons.

We advocate cardiovascular screening of patients with symptoms suggestive of ischaemic heart disease, patients with diabetes mellitus, patients older than 70 years. The tests used will vary as above but exercise ECG testing or exercise thallium scanning are widely used. Patients with positive tests should be referred for cardiological opinion and /or revascularisation where appropriate prior to renal transplantation.

Obesity increases surgical risk and a body mass index (BMI) or 35 or more is often used as a cut-off for suitability for renal transplantation.

Previous malignancy excludes patients unless 5 years have elapsed without evidence of recurrence. The exception is non-melanomatous, non-metastatic skin cancer which does not preclude transplantation but patients should be counselled about the increased risk of skin cancer after transplantation in general.

Medications that may alter calcineurin inhibitor blood concentration or have hazardous interactions

ACEI	increased risk of hyperkalaemia
Allopurinol	possibly increases plasma concentration of CsA

Amiodarone	NB Inhibits metabolism of azathioprine: dose of aza must be drastically reduced possible increase plasma ciclosporin concentation
Macrolides	increase plasma CsA concentration
Rifampicin	reduces plasma CsA concentration
Antiepileptics	decrease plasma CsA concentration
Antifungals	increase plasma CsA concentration
Antimalarials	increase plasma CsA concentration
CCB	increase CsA plasma concentration (specially non-dihydropyridine CCB eg diltiazem)
Cimetidine	possibly increases CsA plasma concentration
Colchicine	increase plasma CsA concentration
Potassium sparing diuretics	risk of hyperkalaemia
Statins	increased risk of myopathy (check CPK)
Tacrolimus	prolong half-life and risk of toxicity

Pneumocystis carinii infection

Co-trimoxazole two 960 mg tablets tds PO for 21 days. Serum therapeutic level (4 hours post dose) for trimethoprim 5–8 mg/L; and for sulphomethoxazole 100–150 mg/L.
I.V dose of co-trimoxazole 120 mg/kg four times/day for 14 days.

Pentamidine isetionate given by IV infusion 4 mg/kg/d IV for at least 14 days (reduce according to product literature in renal impairment) is an alternative for patients who cannot tolerate co-trimoxazole, or who have not responded to it.

Pneumonia in renal transplant recipient

Early microbiological diagnosis (including sputum and blood cultures, broncho-alveolar-lavages etc), reduction of the immunosuppressive therapy and prompt administration of antibiotics are essential in the management of severe pneumonia in renal transplant recipient.

Initiate empirical antibiotic therapy with erythromycin 250–500 mg qds PO or clarithromycin 250–500 mg bd PO or Augmentin 375–

625 tds PO. Keep a close eye on cyclosporin blood level! Add trimethoprim-sulfamethoxazole if infection is severe. Within the next 48 hours switch the therapy to proper antibiotics according to the results of sensitivity testing.

Post transplant lymphoproliferative disease (PTLD)

Discontinue azathioprine or mycophenolate mofetil.
Reduce Prednisolone to 7.5–10 mg/day.
Reduce cyclosporine (or tacrolimus) by 20% every two weeks and discontinue (important) when approximately 30% of the initial dose was reached.

Treatments used in very small number of patients include: monoclonal antibodies, interferon alpha, Ganciclovir or Acyclovir, autologous lymphokine activated killer cells.

PTLD is not contraindication to re-transplantation after complete remission has been obtained and there is no laboratory evidence of active viral replication in the blood. Quantitative PCR for EBV should be used to monitor viral load regularly.

Post-transplant erythrocytosis

Low doses of ACE inhibitors (Enalapril 2.5 mg OD; Lisinopril 5 mg PO od) or angiotensin II receptor inhibitor are effective. In some patients venesection may be required.

Postoperative fluid volume replacement

Fluid replacement with normal saline and 5% dextrose in proportions 2:1.
Volume of the replacement fluid is related to central venous pressure:
CVP >15: give the volume equivalent of previous hour urine output;
CVP 10–15: give the volume equivalent of previous hour urine output plus 30 ml;
CVP 5–10: give the volume equivalent of previous hour urine output plus 70 ml;
CVP less than 5: give the volume equivalent of previous hour urine output plus 70 ml plus 250 ml colloid solution.
Stop IV fluid replacement on day 3 or 4 when urine output is adequate.

Check serum potassium at least twice daily if urine output is massive and adjust replacement (include 20–40 mmol/L potassium with replacement fluid).

Pregnancy

Steroids, azathioprine at doses of 2 mg/kg/day and cyclosporin are safe in pregnancy.
There are not sufficient data on the safety of Tacrolimus in pregnancy.
Cyclosporin and Tacrolimus (if used) metabolism are altered in pregnancy and the blood level therefore should be frequently checked.
Mycophenolate mofetil should be discontinued 6 weeks before conception is attempted.
In the perinatal period the steroid dose should be augmented.
Hydrocortisone 100 mg four times a day should be given during labour and delivery.
Vaginal delivery is recommended in most transplant recipient women.

Surgery (non-transplant related)

On the day of operation the dose of steroids should be augmented, instead of oral prednisolone use IV hydrocortisone 100 mg 3–4 times/day. If it is not possible to take orally, give cyclosporin IV 1/3 of daily oral dose.

The maintenance dose of steroids can be resumed on the second post-operative day.

Perioperative antibiotic prophylaxis to reduce the risk of wound infection with antibiotics directed against skin pathogens and urinary tract infection pathogens: Vancomycin 1 g slow IV over 100 min plus Cephalexin 250 mg qds PO or 500 mg bd PO.

Other antibiotics that may be used: cephalosporins, quinolones, beta-lactams.
Antibiotics should be administered perioperatively and discontinued after 2–3 days after operation to minimize the risk of resistant microorganism growth.

Thrombotic thrombocytopaenic purpura (TTP) and haemolytic uraemic syndrome (HUS)

Both cyclosporine and tacrolimus may produce glomerular thrombotic lesions (thrombotic microangiopathy) similar to TTP or HUS. Therefore stop calcineurin inhibitor and treat the patient with mycophenolate mofetil and prednisolone. Plasma exchange and plasma infusions are also used in the treatment of these conditions.

Tuberculosis (TB) prophylaxis

Patients who are PPD positive pre-transplantation should receive prophylaxis with Isoniazid 300 mg once daily for 6–12 months after transplant operation. Reduce the dose of isoniazid to 200 mg od PO if serum creatinine>300 mmol/L. The drug can cause hepatotoxicity; therefore check liver function. Pyridoxine (vitamin B6) 10 mg PO od is usually co-administered to prevent peripheral neuropathy.

Tuberculosis treatment

With the increase of multidrug-resistant strains therapy should include a minimum of four antituberculous drugs until sensitivities are known.
Initial therapy (2 months):
Isoniazid (INH)
Rifampicin
Pyrazinamide
Ethambutol
Of these, at least two drugs should be continued for an additional 4–10 months according to sensitivity results. Therapy should last for a total of 12 months.
Isoniazid and rifampicin affect calcineurin inhibitor level; isoniazid increases and rifampicin lowers CsA or tacrolimus blood concentration. Therefore monitoring of the level of calcineurin inhibitors 1–3 days after starting antitiberculous therapy is necessary and dosage adjustment is required. In relation to hepatotoxicity isoniazid is the most toxic, therefore monitoring of liver enzymes is required.

Urinary tract infections

The typical microorganisms causing posttransplant UTI are the enteric gram-negative bacilli and enterococci. Midstream urine culture and antibiogram should guide the therapy.

In the early post-transplant period even low bacterial count in the urine (10^2) should be treated. Treatment for early in-hospital UTI and all UTIs associated with bacteraemia or pyelonephritis should begin with parenteral antimicrobials until the urine cultures are negative; oral agents, based upon the sensitivity of the organisms, are then continued for two to six weeks.

UTI developing 3 months after transplantation should be treated for 4–6 weeks. Later 10 – 14 days course is recommended.

Recurrent infections (pyelonephritis) should be treated for 3 weeks.

UTIs developing more than three to six months after transplantation are usually more benign and are clinically indistinguishable from UTIs in the general population. In the absence of pyelonephritis or bacteraemia, they can be treated with a conventional 10 to 14 day course of oral antibiotics. Frequent recurrences require urological evaluation. Native kidneys as a site of infection should also be considered. Most often used drugs are Trimethoprim-sulphomethoxazole 480 mg bd PO or 960 mg PO at bedtime or Ciprofloxacin 250 mg bd PO.

Prophylactic co-trimoxazole has become standard for the first 3–6 months (some groups administer this for 1 year) after transplantation (not only for Pneumocystis carini but also for UTI). The dose of co-trimoxazole should be adjusted according to renal function: 960 mg tablet daily if the plasma creatinine concentration is less than 3 mg/dL (265 μmol/L), and one 960 mg every other day or a 480 mg tablet daily if the plasma creatinine concentration is greater than 3 mg/dL (>265 μmol/L). Patients who are allergic to trimethoprim-sulfamethoxazole can use any of the oral quinolones (ciprofloxacin) for prophylaxis of urinary tract infection.

Indefinite therapy is indicated in patients with a history of recurrent UTIs, anatomical urinary tract abnormalities or other high-risk patients.

More details on Urinary tract infections under separate headings.

Ureteric stent and ureteral catheter

Routine policy is for ureteric anastomosis to be stented. Stent should be removed at about 6 weeks by flexible cystoscopy – the procedure being covered by ciprofloxacin 200 mg PO 1 hour before intervention.

Urine bladder catheter is usually removed on day 5.

Varicella/zoster infection

Prophylaxis: Acyclovir 600 mg/day in divided doses until 6 months post transplantation.

If immunocompromised patient with no detectable VZV antibodies comes into contact with VZ patient, zoster immune globulin (ZIG) should be administered.

Therapy of Varicella infection:
Normal renal function: Acyclovir 10 mg/kg IV every 8 hours for 7–10 days
GFR 10–50 ml/min: Acyclovir 10 mg/kg IV every 12–24 hours
GFR <10 ml/min: Acyclovir 10 mg/kg every 24 hours

Therapy of Herpes zoster:
Normal renal function: Valacyclovir 1 g tds or Acyclovir 800 mg five times a day for 7 days.

Vaccinations

Live virus vaccines are contraindicated post-transplantation.

Withdrawal of immunosuppression after renal transplant failure

In early allograft failure (less than 1 year after transplantation) immediate withdrawal of immunosuppression combined with preemptive nephrectomy.

In patients with renal transplant failure more than one year after transplantation and who return to dialysis, withdraw calcineurin inhibitors (cyclosporine or tacrolimus) and azathioprine or mycophenolate mofetil and taper steroids gradually by 1 mg/month. Some centers reduce calcineurin inhibitors gradually.

TUMOUR LYSIS SYNDROME

Metabolic complications of rapidly growing neoplasms or of the treatment of malignancy that require prophylaxis or treatment are:

Acute renal failure
Hyperuricaemia
Hyperphosphataemia

Hyperkalaemia
Hypocalcaemia

Prophylaxis of these complications include:

Allopurinol should be given to all patients with acute myeloid leukaemia in a dose of at least 300 mg/day PO as soon as the diagnosis is established in order that chemotherapy can be administered as soon as is medically appropriate. In the presence of hyperuricaemia and/or increased cellular turnover, a starting dose of 600 mg/day PO should be considered. Allopurinol should be given for at least 2 days prior to chemotherapy in high doses of 600 – 900 mg daily in divided doses.

In most patients, urate nephropathy can be avoided or ameliorated with vigorous hydration using isotonic saline up to 2.5 litres per day IV and loop diuretic (possibly mannitol), urinary alkalinization with systemic or oral administration of sodium bicarbonate (caution in patients with hyperphosphataemia).

Allopurinol can usually be discontinued within a day or two after chemotherapy is completed.

More rapid declines in uric acid levels are seen following the intravenous administration of rasburicase as IV infusion 200 micrograms/kg once daily for 5 – 7 days. It may be particularly valuable in patients with rapidly growing malignancies associated with hyperuricaemia and tumour lysis syndrome.

Therapy of acute renal failure in patients with tumour lysis syndrome:

- Allopurinol 300 mg od PO
- Loop diuretic (to promote diuresis)
- Sodium bicarbonate has no effect at this stage.
- Haemodialysis should be used if diuresis can not be induced; it is very efficient in removing an excess of uric acid and phosphate.
- Peritoneal dialysis is much less effective than haemodialysis in removing the excess of uric acid.
- Continuous arterio-venous haemodialysis and continuous veno-venous haemofiltration may be used as well in treating ARF due to tumour lysis.

UPPER GASTROINTESTINAL TRACT HEMORRHAGE

Insert peripheral intravenous cannula.
Take blood for: FBC, prothrombin time, U&E/creatinine, x - match 2–6 units of whole blood.
If patient is not hypovolaemic infuse 5% dextrose slowly
If hypovolaemic (pulse >100/min, systolic blood pressure <100 mmHg and/or postural hypotension) infuse Haemacccel stat (max 2 units, or 2x500 ml) then crystalloid and change to blood as soon as possible.
If hypovolaemic, Hb <10 g/L, transfuse (1 unit of blood = 1 g of Hgb)
Correct coagulation deficit: Vit K 10 mg slowly IV in 5% dextrose od or FFP
Insert central venous line for checking CVP.
Endoscopy as soon as possible. Keep nil by mouth until endoscopy.
Gastroscopy should be done within 24 hours, especially if the patient needs more than 4 units of blood and if the patient is >65 years of age.

URINARY TRACT INFECTIONS

(See also Pregnancy, Renal transplant)

Take complete urine analysis and culture before starting antibiotics. Adjust antibiotics to culture results (antimicrobial drug sensitivity).

Asymptomatic bacteriuria (5–10 WBC/HPF or >10^3 microorganisms/mL)

Selected high-risk patients (pregnant women in second or third trimester, renal transplant or patients with neutropenia) may benefit from treatment of asymptomatic bacteriuria. Otherwise, treatment of asymptomatic bacteriuria in general population seems unwarranted and may result in more resistant microorganisms.
Pregnant women should be treated for 7 days (See Pregnancy – Urinary tract infections).

Symptomatic pyuria without bacteriuria

In an otherwise healthy sexually active young person suggests chlamydial or gonococcal urethritis. After confirmation of diagnosis either a single dose of azithromycin 1 g PO) or a 7-day course of doxycycline (100 mg bd PO) is effective for chlamydial urethritis. Therapy of gonococcal urethritis includes a single dose of ceftriaxone (single dose 250 mg IM) or a fluoroquinolone (single dose ciprofloxacin 500 mg PO) combined with doxycycline.

Treatment of uncomplicated UTI

Cystitis: standard therapy is 3 days short course of trimethoprim 200 mg bd PO (or trimethoprim-sulfamethoxazole 960 mg bd PO only when there is good bacterial sensitivity to TMP/SMX) or ciprofloxacin 250 mg bd PO for 3 days if uropathogens resistant to TMP.

If despite treatment symptoms persist or worsen, do a urine culture and prescribe antibiotics according to the results of the culture and sensitivity tests.

Amoxicillin has replaced ampicillin; it is less effective in three-day regimen unless enterococcus is found to be aetiologic agent.

Nitrofurantoin is active against many uropathogens in non-complicated UTI 100 mg bd PO for 7 days. Patients with Cr.cl <60 ml/min should not receive this drug.

Seven-days regimen of therapy for cystitis should be reserved for patients with complicating factors (diabetes, repeated infections)

Complicated UTI

Patients with systemic signs of an acute UTI (flank pain, fever, disuria) or with pyuria and $>10^5$ microorganisms/ml, and who may require IV therapy should be admitted and if gram negative bacilli are seen on microscopical examination give a single IV dose of gentamicin 5 mg/kg/d IV plus followed by fluoroquinolone (ciprofloxacin 500 mg bd PO).

Fluoroquinolone (Ciprofloxacin) could be administered IV (pending on sensitivity) at a dose of 400 mg bd .

For pseudomonas aeruginosa infections:
- Ceftazidime 1 g tds IV or 2 g bd IV or
- Meropenem 500 mg tds IV or
- quinolones (Levofloxacin 500 mg od or bd for 7–14 days)

If gram-positive cocci are seen in the urine ampicillin 1 g every 4 h, or amoxicillin/clavulanate (Augmentin 500/125 tds PO).

The medication should be adjusted if necessary after receiving the result of urine culture. If urine culture is not available after 24 hours, and patient is still symptomatic, continue with reduced dose of gentamicin and keep oral ciprofloxacin as before. 14 days of antimicrobial therapy is appropriate.

If patient has sepsis or septic shock, IV fluid must be given to maintain adequate tissue perfusion which usually results in urine output of >50 ml/h. Antibiotics in sepsis (urosepsis): potential gram-negative pathogens are generally covered with two effective agents from different antibiotic classes, usually beta-lactam (Meropenem 1 g IV every 8 h as a 5 min bolus) + aminoglycoside Gentamicin 3 mg/kg/d IV (check blood level, trough level should be <2 mg/L). Aminoglycoside could be substituted by Ciprofloxacin 200 – 400 mg bd IV or PO.

The other option is a third generation cephalosporin such as Ceftriaxone 1 g od IV, Cefotaxime 2x1 g IV, ceftazidime 1–2 g bd IV or Cefuroxime 1.5 g tds IV.

Fluoroqinolones should not be used in pregnancy or in children.

Parenteral beta-lactams are reserved for more complicated infections: Ceftriaxone 1 g/d IM or IV over 2–4 min; Ceftazidime 1 g bd IM or IV has also good activity against gram-negative bacteria including Pseudomonas aeruginosa.

Continuous prophylaxis

Currently recommended continuous prophylaxis for patients after eradication of an acute infection include:
- Trimethoprim/sulphamethoxazole 480 mg at bedtime or
- Trimethoprim 100 mg at bedtime or
- Nitrofurantoin 50 – 100 mg PO at bed time

VASCULAR ACCESS (a-v fistula, central venous catheter-"line", a-v graft)

Access thrombosis

Prevention of access thrombosis: avoid hypovolaemia, hypotension, identify early venous stenosis (by blood flow monitoring) and if it is diagnosed do percutaneous transluminal angioplasty even before thrombectomy would be needed.

If thrombosis develops - discuss de-clotting with radiologist or surgeons.
Aspirin is of no effect in preventing a-v access thrombosis. There are no definite nor conclusive clinical trials on the positive effect in prevention of access thrombosis by Dipyridamole, ACEI, fish oil, statins, CCB.

Blocked permcath catheter: flush with boluses of 30 ml saline; if ineffective try urokinase or alteplase. Dilute urokinase 5000 units/vial with normal saline. The added volume of saline should be the total volume of both permcath lumens. Instill urokinase in each permcath lumen and clamp permcath. After 30 min aspirate urokinase lock and try haemodialysis. If unsuccessful repeat the procedure three times. Systemic urokinase is more effective and should be tried if lock does not work

Protocol with alteplase: instill 1 mg/ml solution, approximately 2 ml into each lumen of permcath. Clamp, leave for 30 min. After 30 min aspirate alteplase and start haemodialysis. If unsuccessful – repeat the procedure three times.

Patients with recurrent thrombosis may benefit from prophylactic Warfarin aiming for an INR 2–2.5.

Any patient who develops a tendency to clotting dialyser or fistula should be put on Aspirin 75 mg od PO.

Poor flow/blocked line: change the line over guidewire.

Catheter/fistula/PDF graft related infection

Infection is a frequent complication and may be life-threatening. Usually it is due to Staphylococcus aureus or Staphylococcus epidermidis. Remove line after taking cultures from the line (and via a peripheral venepuncture). Start empirical therapy with Vancomycin

1 g in 100 ml saline over 1 hour, then Flucloxacillin 1 g qds IV. Continue antibiotic according to sensitivity for at least 7 days after line removal. This will usually be Flucloxacillin 500 mg qds. Infection of PDF grafts requires admission and treatment with IV antibiotics. PDF graft may need resection. Treat fistula infection as for bacterial endocarditis, i.e. antibiotics for 6 weeks.
Dressing with dry, not-transparent gauze
Mupirocin at catheter exit site
Lock catheter with Gentamicin/citrate
Risk reduction of access infection may be achieved by nasal administration of Mupirocin.

VASCULITIS

Initial therapy (remission induction) requires high-dose cyclophosphamide and corticosteroids, with additional therapy (pulse doses of methylprednisolone and cyclophosphamide and plasmapheresis) in those with life-threatening or organ-threatening disease. In those with non-organ-threatening renal involvement (creatinine <5.6 mg/100 ml; or <500 µmol/L), a commonly used approach is prednisolone 1 mg/kg od PO to a maximum of 80 mg/d, with reducing doses over time to 12.5 – 15 mg by 3 month and cyclophosphamide 2.5 mg/kg/d, adjusted for age (2 mg/kg/d for >70 years of age), renal function, and the white cell count. Cyclophosphamide is maintained for 3 months, and followed by azathioprine (See below Remission maintenance)

As long as steroid dose >10 mg/d routinely give ranitidine 150 mg po BD or Omeprazole 20 mg po OD for gastric protection; Amphotericin B 1 lozenge per day or Nystatin 100,000 u qds PO for fungal prophylaxis and co-trimoxazole 480 mg three times a week for prophylaxis of Pneumocystis carinii, Nocardia and nasal Staphylococcus aureus.

Monitor WBC weekly; stop cyclophosphamide if total WBC <3.5×10^9/l or neutrophil count < 2.0×10^9/l. When WBC has recovered restart cyclophosphamide at 75% of previous dose.

Reduce prednisolone progressively: for example assuming starting dose of 60 mg daily (time 0) reduce to 45 mg daily at two weeks, to 30 mg daily at four weeks then by 5 mg at two weekly intervals down to 10 mg daily at 12 weeks. Continue prednisolone 10 mg daily.

Vasculitis protocol for severely ill patients:

Patients who present with fulminant disease require intensification of induction therapy with the addition of methylprednisolone and/or plasma exchange. A recent European trial indicated that plasma exchange is superior to methylprednisolone in such patients: the effect of combining both approaches has not yet been tested.

Methylprednisolone pulse doses 500 mg IV (if b.w. <75 kg) or 1 g IV (if b.w. >75 kg), in 100 ml isotonic saline over 1 hr for 3 consecutive days. After IV steroids continue with oral, i.e. Prednisolone 0.85 mg/kg/day from day 4. Reduce dose to 0.65 mg/kg/day from day 14. Reduce dose to 0.5 mg/kg/day from the end of week 6. Reduce the dose to 0.3 mg/kg/day from week 12. Reduce the dose to 0.2 mg/kg/day from week 21. Reduce the dose to 0.15 mg/kg/day from week 28. Reduce the dose to 0.07 mg/kg/day from week 36. Stop after one year of therapy.

Plasma exchange for dialysis dependent patients or those with other life-threatening organ involvement, i.e. severe pulmonary hemorrhage: at least 7 exchanges, every other day, each exchange 60 ml/kg, volume of exchange maximum 4 Liters, substitute fluid ½ (50%) 4.5% albumin, ½ (50%) fresh frozen plasma.

Remission maintenance: Therapy with cyclophosphamide should continue for up to three months, at three months, assuming clinical remission, stop cyclophosphamide and replace with azathioprine. Continue the maintenance therapy with azathioprine 2–3 mg/kg/day initially, reducing to 1.5 mg/kg/day by the end of the first year. Duration of therapy with azathioprine is at least one year.

Assess disease activity clinically (symptoms and signs), ANCA, CRP and renal function. Most people enter remission within 4–6 weeks, ideally becoming ANCA negative. More recently, mycophenolate mofetil (MMF) has been used as an alternative to azathioprine.

Check WBC and liver function monthly.

After one year, if clinically in remission and ANCA negative, consider slowly reducing and stopping both azathioprine and prednisolone. Some groups maintain long-term low doses of both azathioprine and prednisolone because of the risk of relapse.

Relapse - minor: increase prednisolone dosage temporarily. Major relapse: conventional management is to restart cyclophosphamide instead of azathioprine. In patients who are intolerant of azathioprine or who relapse whilst taking it, Mycophenolate mofetil could be administered starting at 250 mg po BD and increasing to 1 g bd over 3–4 weeks.

Alternative strategies in a group of patients that frequently relapse or already have the high cumulative dose of cyclophosphamide could be the use of tumour necrosis factor (TNF) blockade, polyclonal antithymocyte globulin (ATG), monoclonal anti-lymphocyte antibodies, or deoxyspergualin.

WATER DEPRIVATION TEST

To diagnose diabetes insipidus, and distinguish it from primary polydipsia. This test assesses the ability of patients to concentrate their urine when fluids are withheld. Water deprivation should normally cause increased secretion of antidiuretic hormone (ADH) resulting in small volumes of concentrated urine. In patients who are clinically water-depleted and/or have hypernatraemia, further fluid restriction may be dangerous.

Unrestricted fluids are allowed overnight. Patients must not eat or drink during the test itself. Close observation of patients is essential to prevent surreptitious /"accidental" drinking and to detect signs of genuine distress due to any rise in plamsa osmolality. Urine should be collected at the bedside.

At 8 am: ask the patient to void urine. Measure urine osmolality (20 ml aliquot of urine) and serum osmolality (5 mls clotted blood). Weigh the patient and record baseline weight.

At 10 am: ask the patient to void urine. Record urine volume. Measure urine osmolality (20 ml aliquot of urine). Weigh the patient and record weight.

At 12 noon: take a further blood sample for serum osmolality. Ask the patient to void urine. Record urine volume. Measure urine osmolality (20 ml aliquot of urine). Weigh the patient and record weight.

At 2pm: ask the patient to void urine. Record urine volume. Measure urine osmolality (20 ml aliquot of urine). Weigh the patient and record weight.

At any other time the patient passes urine, record the time and urine volume and keep a 20 ml sample to measure urine osmolality.

At 4 pm: end the test. Ask the patient to void urine. Record urine volume. Measure urine osmolality (20 ml aliquot of urine). Weigh the patient and record weight. Take a further blood sample for serum osmolality.

N.B. Stop the test at any point if the patient's weight has decreased by more than 5% of baseline body weight or the serum osmolality rises above 300 mOsmols/kg. The test may also be stopped if urine osmolality rises above 700 mOsmols/kg as further water deprivation would not yield any additional information.

Interpretation: If the maximum urine osmolality is above 700 mOsmols/kg, the renal concentrating power is normal and diabetes insipidus is excluded. If the urine osmolality remains below 400 mOsmols/kg throughout the test and the serum osmolality is raised, an inability to concetrate the urine is demonstrated. This supports a diagnosis of diabetes insipidus, DI (although it can also be due to renal tubular disease, this should be evident from other clinical features. DI is diagnosed in the absence of any evidence of renal tubular disease). To distinguish cranial DI from nephrogenic DI, a DDAVP test should be performed (see below).

In primary polydipsia, the urine is usually adequately concentrated (osmolality above 700 mOsmols/kg) and serum osmolality only rises slightly in response to water deprivation. However, an intermediate result (ie urine osmolality between 400 and 700) may occur due to a "washout effect" resulting in loss of medullary concentrating ability.

If the serum osmolality drops and/or the body weight rises during the test, it is very likely that the patient has covertly ingested fluid during the test period.

DDAVP test: this is to distinguish between cranial DI (lack of ADH) and nephrogenic DI (resistance to the action of ADH). The water deprivation test is repeated as above, then at 4pm if the urine osmolality remains below 700 mOsmols/kg, proceed to DDAVP test. At 5 pm (Day 1) the patient is given 20 micrograms of desmopressin (DDAVP) intranasally (or alternatively 0.2 microgram IM). The fluid fast can then be broken, but total fluid intake should be restricted to 1000 ml until 9 am the next morning (Day 2) unless the patient's weight loss exceeds 1.5 kg, when free fluids can be allowed.

At 9 pm and 12 midnight of Day 1 and at 9 am of Day 2 ask the patient to void urine. At these times, and at any other time that the patient voids urine, measure urine osmolality on a 20 ml aliquot of urine, record the urine volume and record the patient's weight.

Interpretation: in cranial DI the urine osmolality should rise above 700 mOsmols/kg. In nephrogenic DI the urine usually fails to concentrate to 700 mOsmols/kg.

BIBLIOGRAPHY

British National Formulary, Pharmaceutical Press, Oxon, UK. ISBN: 0 85369 465 6

Comprehensive guide to prescribing including an excellent section on Prescribing in Renal impairment.

Evidence-based recommendations for the management of glomerulonephritis. Kidney International Supplement 1999 June; volume 70.

Set of articles reviewing evidence base for management of glomerulonephritis.

Kamesh L, Harper L, Savage OC. ANCA-Positive Vasculitis. J Am Soc Nephrol 2002;13:1953–1960.

Extensive review of therapy of vasculitis.

Sprigings D, Chambers J. Acute Medicine. Third Edition, Blackwell Science2001;344–348.

Hyperkalemia

De Vriese A S, Prevention and treatment of acute renal failure in sepsis. J Am Soc Nephrol 2003;14:792–805.

Sepsis and septic shock

Rose BD (Editor-in-Chief), UpToDate, 34 Washington Street, Wellesley, MA 02481, USA.

The clinical reference on CD-ROM and on-line for Nephrology and other subspecialties.

INDEX

Access, Vascular 130
Acetaminophen, poisoning (see Paracetamol) 84
Acidosis 1
Acutely Disturbed Patient 1
Acute Renal Failure 2
Adult Polycystic Kidney Disease 4
Analgaesics 6
Anaphylactic Shock 7
Anticoagulation 8
Antiphospholipid Antibody Syndrome 11
Ascites 12
Athero-embolism (See Cholesterol Crystal Atheroembolic
Renal Disease) 24
Atrial Fibrillation 12
Bacterial Endocarditis 14
Bladder Catheterisation 14
Body Surface Area 14
Bradycardia 15
Candidiasis 15
CAPD 16
Carpal Tunnel Syndrome 23
Cellulitis 23
Cerebral Oedema 24
Cholesterol Crystal Atheroembolic Renal Disease 24
Cholesterol Embolism (see Cholesterol Crystal Atheroembolic
Renal Disease) 24
Chronic Renal Failure, drug prescription 40
Chronic Renal Insufficiency 25
Clostridium difficile Diarrhoea 31
Colic (renal) 32
Contrast Induced Nephropathy 32
Corticosteroids 33
Cramps, muscular 33
Cryoglobulinaemia, mixed 80

Deep Venous Thrombosis & Pulmonary Embolism 34
(see Anticoagulation page 8)
Dental & Minor Surgical Procedures 79
Depression 34
Diabetes Mellitus 34
Disturbed Patient, acute 1
Diuretics 39
Drug Prescription in Chronic Renal Failure 40
Eclampsia 46
Embolism, pulmonary 34
Endocarditis, bacterial 14
Epilepsy 46
Erectile Dysfunction 46
Ethylene Glycol Intoxication 47
Fibrosis, Retroperitoneal 96
Fluid (for IV administration) 47
Glomerular Filtration Rate 49
Glomerulonephritis 50
Haemodialysis 56
Haemolytic Uraemic Syndrome 106
Haemorrhage, upper gastrointestinal tract 127
Helicobacter Pylori, eradication of 86
Hepatitis B 64
Hepatitis C 65
Hepato-Renal Syndrome 66
Hiccups 67
Hypercalcaemia 67
Hyperhomocysteinaemia 68
Hyperkalaemia 68
Hypernatraemia 69
Hyperprolactinaemia 69
Hypertension 70
Hypocalcaemia 75
Hypokalaemia 75
Hyponatraemia 76
Influenza 76
Insomnia 76
Inotropes 77
Interstitial Nephritis 77
IV Immunoglobulins 78
Legionella Infection 78

Leptospirosis 78
Lupus (see Systemic Lupus Erythematosus) 101
Meningitis 78
Mesna 78
Metabolic Acidosis, in Chronic Renal Failure 1
Methanol Intoxication 79
Minor Surgical & Dental Procedures 79
Mixed Cryoglobulinaemia 80
Muscle Cramps 33
Nasal Screening for Dialysis Patients 81
Nausea and Vomiting 81
Nephrotic Syndrome 82
Neutropaenic Patients 83
Nutrition (oral/tube feeding/parenteral) 84
Oedema, cerebral 24
Paracetamol (acetaminophen) Poisoning 84
Peptic Ulcer & Eradication of Helicobacter Pylori 86
Perioperative Management
(of patients with CRF/renal replacement) 87
Plasmapheresis 89
Pneumonia 90
Poisoning, paracetamol 84
Polycystic Kidney Disease, adult 4
Pulmonary embolism 34
Purpura
(see Thrombotic Thrombocyopaenic Purpura &
Haemolytic Uraemic Syndrome) 106
Pregnancy 90
Renal Artery Stenosis 96
Renal Colic 32
Renal Transplantation 106
Retroperitoneal Fibrosis 96
Rhabdomyolysis 97
Sepsis and Septic Shock 98
Shock, anaphylactic 7
Shock, septic 98
Stenosis, Renal Artery 96
Systemic Lupus Erythematosus 101
Thrombotic Thrombocytopaenic Purpura
& Haemolytic Uraemic Syndrome 106
Transplantation (Renal) 106

Tumour Lysis Syndrome.. 125
Upper Gastrointestinal Tract Haemorrhage.................................... 127
Urinary Tract Infections 127
Vascular Access 130
Vasculitis.. 131
Vomiting, Nausea and.. 81
Water Deprivation Test 133

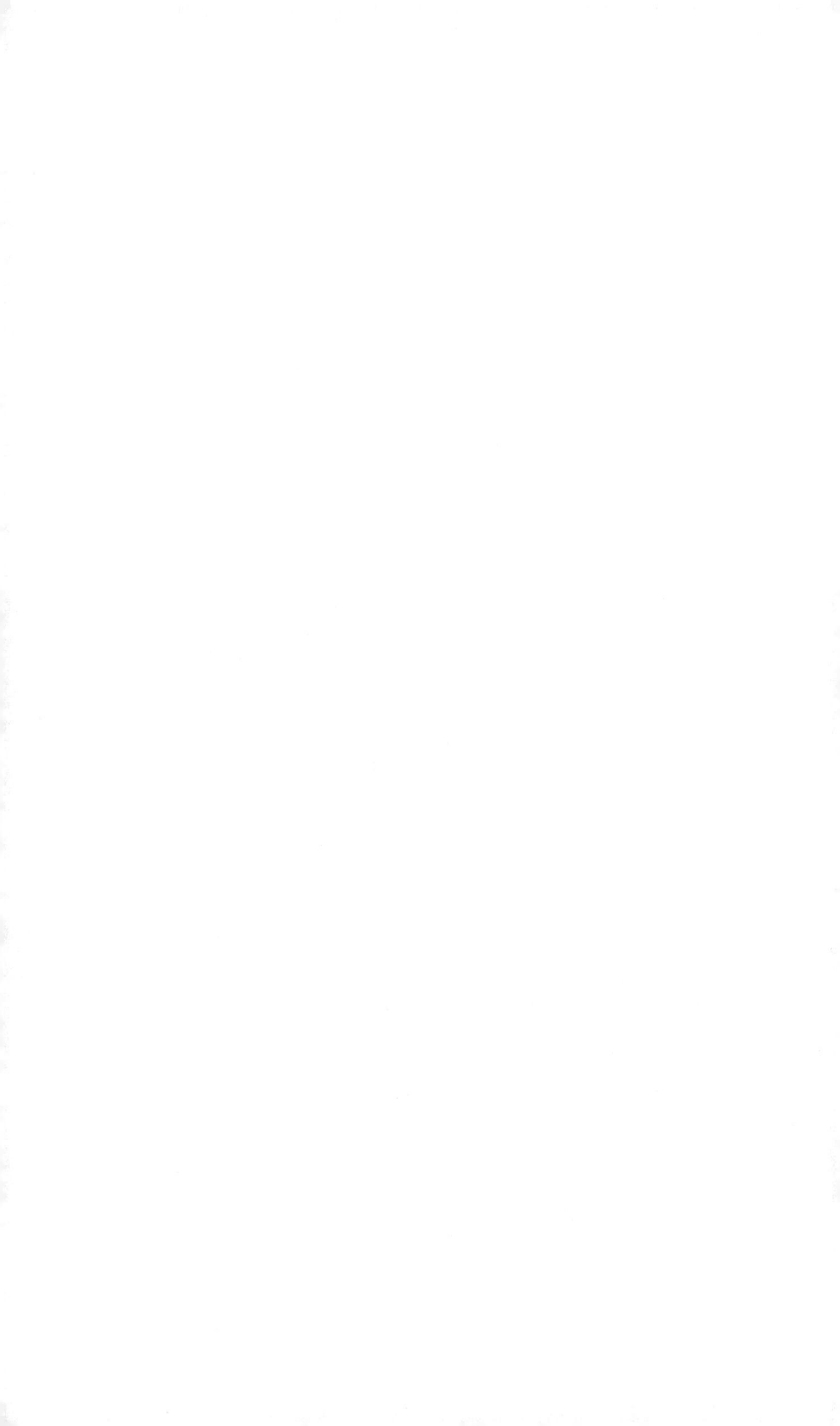

www.ingramcontent.com/pod-product-compliance
Lightning Source LLC
Chambersburg PA
CBHW030755180526
45163CB00003B/1033